Praise for *Drop the Disorder!*

Anyone who wants to deal with the epidemic of distress and despair in our society should engage deeply with Jo Watson's work and this massively important book.
Johann Hari, journalist and writer; author of *Lost Connections: why you're depressed and how to find hope*

Drop the Disorder! assembles a group of cutting-edge contributors to shine a light on some of the most contested issues of modern psychiatric practice. Challenging, insightful and often controversial, their perspectives combine rigorous scholarship with the power of lived experience to create a truly innovative and valuable book that functions both as a learning resource and an ardent call to arms. On reaching the end your instinct will almost certainly be to re-read it in order to appreciate its insights for a second time.
Dr Eleanor Longden, Service User Research Manager, Psychosis Research Unit, Greater Manchester Mental Health NHS Foundation Trust

After finishing this brilliant collection of essays, readers will not only agree with the call to 'Drop the Disorder!' but also understand, with great clarity, why it is imperative that psychiatry's *Diagnostic and Statistical Manual (DSM)* be dumped, as quickly as possible, into the waste bin. The *DSM* has been used to tell people that they are suffering from 'diseases' of the brain, with the psychiatric profession then poised to treat those 'diseases'. Upon close inspection, which is what this collection of well-written essays provides, readers will see that the *DSM* is properly seen as a manual promoting what could fairly be called a medical 'delusion'. As such, *Drop the Disorder!* provides a clarion call for change.
Robert Whitaker, author of *Mad in America* **and** *Anatomy of an Epidemic,* **and founder of madinamerica.com**

We live in an age when where being diagnosed with 'mental illness' is a common occurrence. Psychiatric drugs are everywhere, and words like 'serotonin' and 'dopamine' have entered everyday language. But do we really have an epidemic of 'mental illness', or is it psychiatry that's gone mad? This book is packed with rich narratives, incisive analysis and powerful critiques of a world where everyday emotions are increasingly seen as disease. If 'mental illness' has touched your life in any way, drop what you're doing and read *Drop the Disorder!*
Indigo Daya, survivor advocate, blogger, speaker, consumer academic, University of Melbourne and human rights advisor, Victorian Mental Illness Awareness Council, Australia

Drop the Disorder!

CHALLENGING THE CULTURE OF PSYCHIATRIC DIAGNOSIS

EDITED BY JO WATSON

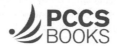

First published 2019

PCCS Books Ltd
Wyastone Business Park
Wyastone Leys
Monmouth
NP25 3SR
contact@pccs-books.co.uk
www.pccs-books.co.uk

Drop the Disorder!
Challenging the culture of psychiatric diagnosis

British Library Cataloguing in Publication data: a catalogue record for this book is
available from the British Library.

ISBN 978 1 910919 46 0

Front cover illustration by Jason Anscomb
Typeset in-house by PCCS Books using Minion Pro and Myriad Pro
Printed by Short Run Press, Exeter, UK

Dedication

Matt Stevenson, I know that you wanted so desperately to stay around and fight for change but you were too deeply and irreparably hurt by psychiatry's labels. This is for you.

Contents

Acknowledgements and thanks

Huge thanks to Pete Sanders and Catherine Jackson at PCCS Books who, since the very first conversations about this book, somehow found an endless supply of encouragement and support and sent it in my direction. And I needed a lot of both! Thanks too to all the PCCS Books team. So much of the work from now will be about getting this book and its message out there.

Thank you to all the chapter contributors for sharing your wisdom and experience. And thank you for all that you do, every day, way beyond your contributions here, to bring about change.

Thank you Gary Sidley, Lanie Pianta and Joanne Newman. The success of the 'Drop the Disorder!' Facebook group is down to your exceptional moderating skills, your total commitment to challenging the bullshit and your capacity to put up with me. Solidarity and love!

Lucy Johnstone, Nollaig McSweeney, Jacqui Dillon and Akima Thomas – thank you for making AD4E such a hopeful and healing experience and for being the best friends and allies.

Thank you, Pat McArdle, my partner in love and life and in the fight to make a difference. *Bean mo chroi – Tiocfaidh ár lá x*

Last, I want to acknowledge the many people I've been honoured to connect with, both personally and professionally, who have shown me over and over again that there is always sense to be made, meaning to be found and stories to be shared.

A note on terminology

A huge part of this book, and, indeed, the challenge to the culture of diagnosis and disorder generally, is about language. Our words have been hijacked; our language has been colonised by biomedical model theory. Western society is fluent in the language of diagnosis and disorder.

Everyday words and phrases that accurately describe human experience – words like sadness, misery, hopelessness, terror, hearing voices, obsessive thoughts, dissociative experience, difficulty, distress, support – have vanished from our vocabularies. Even grief, as Pete Sanders points out in his chapter, has come to be classified as a medical condition.

Instead, we speak and think of human emotions and experiences in diagnostic terms and medicalised words that come straight from biological psychiatry: 'depressive disorder', 'anxiety disorder', 'schizophrenia', 'psychosis', 'symptom', 'treatment', 'illness', 'condition', 'disorder'…

This medicalised lexicon has become so much a part of our language and way of thinking about our feelings and emotions that it would be next to impossible to produce a book about all of this without using these same words that these chapters decry.

With this in mind, I made the decision to use quotation marks around medicalised words and phrases in order to identify them as such to the reader. That said, the majority of authors were doing this anyway to signify their discomfort with using medicalised language.

Quotation marks are used around all diagnostic and medicalised words, including *DSM* diagnoses and words that are closely associated with such diagnoses, such as 'psychosis'. There are no quotation marks around the words 'depression' and 'anxiety' when they are contextualised and used in a lay sense, although I acknowledge that these words are also closely associated with diagnostic categories.

I hope that the consistent use of quotation marks throughout this book will serve to remind the reader that these words represent unscientific constructs and not legitimate medical 'illnesses'.

Jacqui Dillon, in her chapter, calls on us to reclaim the language of human experience from medical colonisation. It's a huge challenge, but I very much hope that this book plays a part in that reclaiming.

Jo Watson

Foreword[1]

Paula J Caplan

Since the mid-1980s, I have done much writing and lecturing to inform people about what I discovered about the classification and treatment of humans' emotional suffering. I was in a unique position, having served on the task force tasked with revising the *Diagnostic and Statistical Manual of Mental Disorders (DSM)*, then resigning on moral, ethical and professional grounds and publicly exposing how the *DSM* leaders make decisions about who is and is not psychologically 'normal'.

As a professor at the University of Toronto, training graduate students in psychology, I had believed the false advertising about the *DSM* that is put out by its publisher, the American Psychiatric Association – that psychiatric diagnostic categories are 1) scientifically based, 2) helpful in reducing human suffering, and 3) not likely to cause harm. When, in 1988, I was invited to serve on two of the committees that would prepare *DSM-IV*, I accepted but said that, if I was not comfortable with what I learned on those committees, I would resign and would feel free to speak publicly about it. That is indeed what happened.

As an insider, privy to internal communications sent to us committee members from committee chairs and from Allen Frances, chair of the *DSM-IV* task force, I learned first that the process of creating psychiatric categories and labels is extremely unscientific. This came as a particular shock but was easy to see because one of my areas of specialisation is research methodology. Given the lack of scientific basis for both their creation and their application, it is

---

1. Part of the crux of this article first appeared on the *Ending Harm from Psychiatric Diagnosis* website (psychdiagnosis.weebly.com), under the title 'Openness/Honesty/Full Disclosure', and readers are urged to read the essay on that website for suggestions about solutions.

no surprise that simply getting one of these labels does not reduce a person's suffering – except perhaps by leading to the misguided and often temporary belief that 'Now I have a label, so now I know what's really causing my trouble, so now the science will show how to fix it'.

I further saw that, when science and objectivity are absent, what of course comes immediately into the process is every conceivable kind of bias and subjectivity. As I spoke out publicly about what I had learned, I began to hear from people whose lives had been ruined in a stunning variety of ways, all of which began with their being psychiatrically labelled. I also learned from them, as well as from my own observation of therapists' discussions of their patients, that once a patient has a label, the range of kinds of help they are offered drastically narrows (nearly always to psychotherapy, psychiatric drugs or both, despite the vast number of helpful and low-risk or no-risk approaches that do not involve calling the person mentally ill[2]), and the therapist's – and other people's – views of the person come to focus on 'what's wrong' with them, while their strengths, resources and existence as a whole person are not even the topics of questions they are asked.

Psychiatric diagnosis is the first cause of everything bad that happens in the mental health system, because if they don't diagnose you, they cannot do *anything* to you, but once they give you *any* of the hundreds of diagnoses, they can do pretty much anything to you in the name of treatment. And, because psychiatric diagnosis is totally unregulated, there is no oversight and little or no recourse for those who are harmed. I was once an expert witness in a lawsuit in which psychotherapists had destroyed a woman's happiness and peace of mind but were not held accountable, on the grounds that what they had done was typical of the 'standard of care'.

Over the decades, I have heard from thousands of people who suffered terribly because of what followed once they were diagnosed – and because they were unaware that their label or labels were unscientific, unlikely to lead to reduction of their suffering and likely to put them at risk for many kinds of harm. The harm ranges from loss of self-confidence to loss of physical health, employment, child custody and the right to make decisions about one's medical and legal affairs – even to loss of life.

When people consider the unscientific nature, lack of helpfulness and frequent harm caused by psychiatric diagnoses, they often nevertheless express alarm about what to do if diagnoses were not used. They often begin with the question, 'What do we call emotional suffering and other problems if we are not going to give them psychiatric labels?' The answer to that is easy. We listen to what people have to tell us, and we apply to their feelings, conflicts and dilemmas the kinds of words that people used before psychiatric labels were created; words

---

2. See www.youtube.com/playlist?list=PL51E99E866B9D735E for more than two dozen examples of such helpful, non-pathologising approaches (accessed 12 June 2019).

the poets and the novelists – and ordinary people – have used; words like *grief, fear, shame, guilt, loneliness, alienation* and *anguish*. We encourage patients to do the same, rather than asking for a diagnosis.

The response to that suggestion is often, 'But those words aren't scientific, so how can they help reduce people's suffering?' The answer to that is: 'Psychiatric labels aren't scientific and do not reduce people's suffering, *and* they put people at great risk of harm.' Furthermore, it makes for a healthier interaction between therapist and patient or between a suffering person and their listening friend or family member when we remove the jargon, mystification and pseudoscience. Indeed, it makes for a healthier society when, in addressing human suffering, we all know what we are talking about.

Drop the Disorder! – as a book and as a movement – is a powerful example of, and force for, this kind of straight, human, humane talk about emotional suffering. Because of this, it helps us see ways that go far beyond the important first step of refusing to use psychiatric diagnoses and leads us to assist people to achieve richer, more interesting, more creative, more connected and more self-determined lives. The chapters in the book represent a stunningly varied and creative collection of incisively educational, artistically brilliant, emotionally moving pieces. Together, they form a prism through which new views of emotional suffering can be seen that reveal its actual causes, reduce the soul-killing treatment of some people as Other, and instead promote health, peace, connection, and delight.

Paula J Caplan
September 2019

Bibliography

Caplan PJ (2005). *The Myth of Women's Masochism*. Lincoln, NE: iUniverse.

Caplan PJ (1995). *They Say You're Crazy: how the world's most powerful psychiatrists decide who's normal*. Reading, MA: Addison-Wesley.

Caplan PJ, Cosgrove L (eds) (2004). *Bias in Psychiatric Diagnosis*. Lanham, MA: Jason Aronson/ Rowman & Littlefield.

Introduction

Jo Watson

'Don't be sorry. Please don't be sorry. Please do something.'
The Handmaid's Tale (Miller, 2017)

In October 2016, Dr Lucy Johnstone and I hosted the very first 'A Disorder for Everyone!' (AD4E) event to explore the culture of psychiatric diagnosis, in Birmingham, UK.

At the same time, to provide a space to continue the debate after the event, I set up the Facebook group 'Drop the Disorder!'

Little did we know that, three years later, along with a group of activist, survivor and professional contributors, we would be returning to Birmingham after visiting cities all over the UK to deliver our 18th AD4E event and launch this book.

The scale of the appetite for discussion about psychiatric diagnosis and the pathologising of emotional distress became clear fairly early on in our AD4E journey. People from all walks of life were attending AD4E events in their hundreds, and expressing their dissatisfaction, frustration and anger with the dominance of the biomedical model in their thousands via the Facebook group, which by its second birthday in September 2018 had more than 8,000 members from all over the world.

This book takes the themes, energy and passions of the AD4E events and the Facebook group discussions and brings together authors from various backgrounds, many of them speakers from the events, to share their stories and deliver their messages in the struggle to bring about change.

My own AD4E journey dates back to early 2016, when my capacity to deal with a culture that relentlessly pathologises people's pain by labelling them as 'disordered' crashed spectacularly, leaving me stuck, frustrated and knowing that

I needed to do something. Many factors – personal, professional and political – played their part in contributing to a peak of despair that, as it turned out, was to be the very catalyst I needed.

Although I can't remember a time when I didn't believe that emotional distress is infinitely more indicative of what has happened in people's lives than of so-called medical diseases and disorders, it was more recently that I started to understand exactly how these diagnoses come to be. I discovered that they are unscientific, made-up constructs voted into existence by the 'opinions' of psychiatrists populating the *Diagnostic and Statistical Manual of Mental Disorders* (*DSM*) committees (Kirk & Kutchins, 1992; Kutchins & Kirk, 1997; Caplan, 1995; Johnstone 2000; Greenberg, 2013; Davies, 2013).

And, given the make-up of the *DSM* committees and the many 'vested interests' around the table (as explained by James Davies in Chapter 6 of this book), I would argue that it is opinion that is highly suspect.

Yet these opinions go on to affect, and sometimes define and control, people's lives. Sometimes their whole lives. The labels put people into boxes and, in too many cases, permanently close the lid, with the words 'life-long conditions'.

So, back in the first couple months of 2016, I became aware of numerous educational establishments referring young people to psychiatric services at the first sign of any expression of distress (self-harm, hearing voices – both normal responses to traumatic experiences). The outcome of these referrals was all too often a psychiatric diagnosis of one 'disorder' or another. Yet in all of the cases that I knew of, there were things happening in the lives of the young person that, in my view, fully explained their distress.

These young people, like millions of others, were sold psychiatry's story that they had a 'mental illness' that needed to be chemically managed. The real stories of what they had experienced were not even acknowledged, let alone linked to the distress.

I could see that more and more people were understanding their own emotional distress through a medicalised lens of 'disorder', because that was the endorsed understanding in the wider world. People had little or no access to any other perspectives. I was also becoming increasingly aware of how the narrative of 'diagnosis' and 'disorder' had managed to infiltrate my own profession of counselling and psychotherapy, as I describe in my chapter.

Around this same time, I read Dr Lucy Johnstone's book *A Straight Talking Introduction to Psychiatric Diagnosis* (Johnstone, 2014), which was a much-needed breath of fresh air and made me feel more hopeful. It also gave me some ideas! I asked Lucy if she was up for being involved in an event based around the core messages of her book. The rest is the story of AD4E.

In *A Straight Talking Introduction to Psychiatric Diagnosis*, Lucy argues that people should have a choice about how they understand their own distress. She suggests we do not *have to* accept diagnostic explanations and proposes other, more helpful ways, of making sense of distress. It is really no exaggeration to say that, over the last few years, I've seen people's lives turned around as a result of reading Lucy's book, simply because it offers alternatives to diagnosis in a really accessible way.

I had always hoped the event in Birmingham would not be a one-off, but I had no idea how fast the momentum would build. Very soon after Birmingham, we had planned our second, third and fourth events in Bristol, Edinburgh and London respectively, and by the time we got to London on 8th June 2017, we'd added Irish activist Nollaig McSweeney to our team, with Dr Jacqui Dillon joining the three of us a little later, further on down the AD4E road.

Meanwhile our list of AD4E speakers was growing fast. As we travelled around the country, we approached inspirational people from a variety of backgrounds who had important things to say. We invited them to speak and we added their biographies to the contributors section of our website. We were collecting allies: activists, authors, academics, survivors, therapeutic professionals, artists, poets and more. As we built these connections, the isolation that I had felt for a long time dissipated and became a distant memory. Support and solidarity, a sense of unity, of togetherness, are crucial. As individuals, fragmented and disconnected from any sense of shared objective, we are powerless; resistance in isolation can so often be futile. Thus, connection with allies is vital; we simply can't afford to be alone. We need to be part of something bigger than us as individuals.

The AD4E events do two main things. First, we challenge the culture of 'diagnosis and disorder'; second, we discuss different ways of understanding distress – ways that are not restricted to the constructs of psychiatry but are about hearing people's stories, making the links with what has happened to them, and making sense of their understandable pain. This by definition takes into account the social contexts that are at the root of so much distress.

All of this is built on the idea of choice, and by that I mean *informed* choice. This, of course, relies on people having the relevant information, and we make no apologies for our attempt to counteract the limitations and biases of the mainstream messages. We offer and we suggest, but we do not impose. People can take the bits they want and leave the bits they don't want.

Offering information about how psychiatric diagnoses are created, what they are and what they aren't, and debunking the myths that are peddled to us by the psychiatric establishment is an important part of what we do. Several chapters in this book contribute to that – not least, those of John Read and Lorenza Magliano, Terry Lynch, James Davies and more. Clare Shaw's chapter tells it powerfully from her personal experience.

Getting the message out is vital and social media have been huge in that. When I launched the 'Drop the Disorder!' Facebook group after the first AD4E event, I expected that a percentage of attendees would join to continue the discussions we had on that day. Maybe 20 or 30? Three years on, and we are fast approaching 10,000 members from all over the world, building up an international movement of allies and resisters.

Twitter and Instagram have been invaluable too. Twitter has allowed us to build more connections and publicise the events; the AD4E Instagram account collects together a wealth of wisdom in the form of quotes, images and memes from allies who have come up with numerous gems of insight and encouragement. Sometimes, when I need a boost, I log on to Instagram and scroll through all the memes of allies' quotes. For me it's a quick shot of hope and solidarity that reminds me I'm not alone and that we are strong in numbers.

Helen Margetts (Margetts et al, 2015), a political scientist at Oxford University, says that social media can make activists of us all. She talks about how social media encourages what she calls 'tiny acts of participation' involving more and more people who can engage simply by liking posts or tweets, signing online petitions, sharing, tweeting, retweeting etc. Every small act of participation on social media equates to a 'digital trace', Margetts argues, and together they add up to large-scale mobilisation. So, there are digital traces of resistance everywhere!

So much else has happened in the last few years, including the launch of Mad in the UK (madintheuk.com), a sister site to www.madinamerica.com, which we were proud to announce at our London event in September 2018. And now, as AD4E approaches its third birthday and 18th event, we continue to be honoured and humbled by people's feedback about how the events have impacted on their lives.

One participant at our Liverpool event said:

> I arrived this morning with a 'mental illness' and I leave knowing that everything I've experienced is an understandable response when I consider all that happened to me as a kid. I am not ill. It makes sense now.

A delegate at our Leeds event said:

> I've never thought this diagnosis stuff fitted with counselling. It doesn't make sense to me as counselling is about hearing someone and diagnosis is pretty much the opposite. Today has given me the encouragement to challenge my organisation about some of the language we are using to describe mental distress as well as the beliefs that may be lingering behind it!

As long as we are receiving this kind of feedback that tells us that lives are being affected in a positive way, it gives us the motivation to keep doing what we are doing. Our skins have undoubtedly had to grow thicker; we've had to deal with personal as well as political attacks and relentless misrepresentation on social media. But, as Terry Lynch so often reminds me: 'They wouldn't bother if what you were doing was irrelevant. Take it as a sign you're having an impact!' We will and we do.

This book is part of that. It emerged from a conversation with Pete Sanders, who has spoken at several AD4E events (and contributes his own chapter here) – a co-founder and director of PCCS Books. He suggested I make this book by drawing together some of the amazing speakers from the events, and others. So I did. My hope is it will carry the energy and passion of its contributors still further afield.

I am grateful to Pete Sanders and PCCS Books for the opportunity to bring together a such an amazing bunch of truth-telling change-makers for whom I have such huge respect.

For me, the energy and passion of people who fight for change are both intoxicating and contagious. In fact, I caught the bug from them a while ago now and, if you're not already afflicted, I'd seriously recommend it as a great bug to catch! (Though, I should warn you, it is, in all probability, a severe, life-long condition.) Unfortunately, there's no 'cure' or 'treatment' as such. However, I've found that it can be 'managed' to some degree by engaging in regular acts of activism and resistance that challenge the culture of pathology.

In the TV adaptation of *The Handmaid's Tale* (Miller, 2017; Atwood, 1996), the main character, June Osborne, risks everything when she tells a visitor about the atrocities that have been happening. The visitor believes her, and says she's sorry but that she can't do anything. June responds: 'Don't be sorry. Please don't be sorry. Please do something.' The truth is that there's little point talking about how damaging the present system is if we are just going to be sorry about it and not do anything.

This book is an unapologetic challenge to the culturally endorsed understanding of emotional distress, and it is a book for everyone. It's for everyone because we all experience such distress and consequently we are all potentially vulnerable to psychiatric diagnosis and what comes from that. It contains academic pieces and personal stories, it offers poetry and metaphor, and it embodies resistance and solidarity. It is, in essence, a call to action.

I hope that your experience of reading it is insightful, affirming and validating. Most of all, I hope that the collective wisdom and courageous sharing in this book will encourage more people to 'do something' to challenge the culture of psychiatric diagnosis and join the struggle to 'drop the disorder!'

Do something

Don't be sorry – Do something!
What? – It doesn't matter
Take your place in the fight back
'cause we've got lies to shatter

Find your thing and do it
Pen ranting rhymes or songs
Meme great quotes for Instagram
Make noise about what's wrong

Wave a banner, share a post
Offer to explain
Plug a book, send a clip
Organise! Campaign!

Write a blog, make a sign
Retweet rage-filled tweets
Join a group, start a group
Fill the bloody streets

Wear a badge, start debates
Talk and rant and shout
Share allies' posts all day long
Giving them more clout

To get the message out there
and smash down all the lies
that dishonour all the stories
and just pathologise

By talking of what's broken
and of illness or condition
sod this game of soldiers
file a petition!

Then get the world to sign it
Let's call the whole thing out
The empire is falling
Not one bit of doubt

Change is around the corner
Their cover has been blown
We know the score, we're fighting back
And we are not alone

There's a world of allies out there
Just waiting to be found
And when we all 'do something'
There'll be a turnaround!

Jo Watson

References

Atwood M (1996). *The Handmaid's Tale*. London: Jonathan Cape.

Caplan PJ (1995). *They Say You're Crazy: how the world's most powerful psychiatrists decide who's normal*. Reading, MA: Addison-Wesley.

Davies J (2013). *Cracked: why psychiatry is doing more harm than good*. London: Icon Books.

Greenberg G (2013). *The Book of Woe: the DSM and the unmaking of psychiatry*. Victoria: Scribe Publications Pty.

Johnstone L (2014). *A Straight Talking Introduction to Psychiatric Diagnosis*. Ross-on-Wye: PCCS Books.

Johnstone L (2000). *Users and Abusers of Psychiatry: a critical look at traditional psychiatric practice* (2nd ed). London: Routledge.

Kirk SA, Kutchins H (1992). *The Selling of DSM: the rhetoric of science in psychiatry*. Hawthorne: Aldine de Gruyter.

Kutchins N, Kirk SA (1997). *Making Us Crazy: DSM: the psychiatric bible and the creation of mental disorders*. New York, NY: The Free Press.

Margetts H, John P, Hale S, Yasseri T (2015). *Political Turbulence: how social media shape collective action*. Princeton, NJ: Princeton University Press.

Miller B (2017). *The Handmaid's Tale*. [TV series.] MGM Television.

1 | Do you still need your psychiatric diagnosis? Critiques and alternatives

Lucy Johnstone

Do you still need your psychiatric diagnosis? A revolution is underway in mental health. If the authors of the diagnostic manuals are admitting that the diagnoses are not supported by evidence and that the process of developing them is not scientifically sound, then no one should be forced to accept them. If many mental health workers are openly questioning diagnosis and saying we need a different and better system, then service users and carers should be allowed to do so too. (Johnstone, 2014).

These words summarise both the themes of my book, *A Straight Talking Introduction to Psychiatric Diagnosis* (Johnstone, 2014), and the series of events, 'A Disorder for Everyone!', that the editor of this book, Jo Watson, and her team have organised across the UK over the last three years. Our shared aim, and that of the many other participants at these events from both professional and survivor backgrounds, is to give people the information to decide whether it makes sense for them to see their problems in diagnostic terms or whether they wish to explore the various alternatives on offer.

In the current UK health and welfare systems, few people can afford to give up diagnosis entirely – it is needed for access to benefits, services etc. But *they may decide they do not wish to define themselves and their problems in this way.* We believe that this decision should be made on the basis of informed choice, and not just a view imposed by a professional. This is also the theme of the chapters in this book.

I will start with a brief summary of the general context and the criticisms of psychiatric diagnosis. This will be followed by an overview of three related alternatives – psychological formulation, the trauma-informed approach and the Power Threat Meaning Framework.

The context of critiques of psychiatric diagnosis

It is important to emphasise that *mental distress is very real.* People undoubtedly do have terrifying and disabling experiences, such as hearing hostile voices, feeling suicidal, being overwhelmed by anxiety, swinging from high to low moods, and so on. What they are very rarely told is that there has never been any evidence to support the dominant explanation for these experiences – in other words, that they are best understood as medical illnesses with primarily biological causes that psychiatric drugs will help to rectify.

This may come as a surprise, since what is referred to as the 'biomedical model' of distress has taken such a hold in public consciousness. Almost every media article, blog, TV programme and anti-stigma campaign makes unquestioning use of language that assumes this perspective – 'bipolar disorder', 'schizophrenia', 'anxiety disorder', 'personality disorder' and, indeed, the term 'mental illness' itself. Few people have failed to hear the message that 'chemical imbalances' are responsible for 'illnesses' such as the experiences we call depression.

In fact, senior psychiatrists are rapidly backtracking on these theories, claiming that '… the "chemical imbalance theory" was never a real theory, nor was it widely propounded by responsible practitioners in the field of psychiatry' (Pies, 2014). Similarly, studies on the likelihood of inheriting what is usually called 'mental illness' have so far failed to come up with any definitive findings at all. Excited headlines about 'genes for schizophrenia' and so on have not yet lived up to their promise. In fact, an objective reading of the evidence shows that by far the largest contribution to distress comes from our environments, supporting the common-sense view that people's emotional wellbeing is negatively affected by poverty, trauma, discrimination, unemployment, loss and the general insecurity of living in an increasingly competitive and unequal society. (For summaries of the debates, see Cromby, Harper & Reavey, 2013; Read & Sanders, 2010; Read & Dillon, 2013.)

Criticisms of psychiatric diagnosis and the biomedical model that it supports are not new. They last came into public awareness in the so-called antipsychiatry movement of the 1960s, in which radical psychiatrist RD Laing and colleagues were key figures. The central message from those days, that madness is meaningful in the context of people's lives and relationships, is as true as it ever was. However, those early critics largely failed to develop coherent alternatives, and mainstream psychiatry has managed to discredit them by labelling them family-blamers, ideologues and extremists (Johnstone, 2018).

Despite this, the controversies have never gone away. What is more, as I hope to show, we now have a range of evidence-based and effective alternatives to the diagnostic approach. Meanwhile, the most unexpected aspect of the current revival of criticisms of diagnosis is that the strongest attacks have come from the world's most senior psychiatrists. In fact, some of them are the very people who were responsible for drawing up the so-called psychiatric bible, the *Diagnostic and Statistical Manual of Mental Disorders*, published by the American Psychiatric Association and now in its fifth edition (APA, 2013), which lists the many ways in which people can be diagnosed as 'mentally ill' or 'disordered'. (The equivalent European manual is called the *International Classification of Diseases* (*ICD*), and is produced by the World Health Organization (2018).) Thus Dr Allen Frances, chair of the *DSM-IV* committee, has openly declared that, 'There is no reason to believe that *DSM-5* is safe or scientifically sound' (Frances, 2013) – although, interestingly, he also claims that the almost identical *DSM-IV* was 'scrupulously scientific' (Frances, 2013). It is important to note that these people are not giving up the diagnostic model. Rather, they are in the tricky position of maintaining that the current unevidenced system is better than nothing, until new ones are developed from scratch.'

The main critiques of psychiatric diagnosis

A brief discussion about what we mean by the process of diagnosing someone with a medical illness will highlight the problems with psychiatric diagnosis.

We may go to our GP to report certain symptoms – thirst, tiredness, nausea and so on. These usually have a strong subjective element and can be present for many reasons. No one can really observe exactly how tired or thirsty you are or how much pain you are in, and obviously there can be many reasons for feeling like this. So, in order to make a diagnosis, the doctor will need to narrow down the range of possible reasons for these complaints by checking for bodily signs, perhaps by running tests. This will, ideally, identify something such as an abnormality in your blood-cell count or levels of sugar in your urine, or some other aspect of bodily functioning that has been shown by medical research to be linked to the symptoms you are experiencing. At this point, the doctor may be able to make a diagnosis of, perhaps, diabetes. Researchers then use this concept as a basis for further research. In some cases, as our knowledge builds up, the original category will be replaced by more accurate terms. For example, we would now refer to 'tuberculosis', rather than 'consumption'. Similarly, in the field of psychiatry, we no longer attribute problems to 'wandering wombs', as was common practice in the Victorian era. Scientific progress depends on constantly revisiting and revising our basic concepts.

The problem with diagnosis in psychiatry is twofold: first, that there are no bodily tests or signs for so-called psychiatric disorders. You cannot have a blood test or a scan for 'schizophrenia' or 'depression'. This means that, in psychiatry, with rare exceptions such as dementia, doctors are stuck at the personal report or 'symptom' level; they can never actually confirm or disconfirm a diagnosis by saying, for example: 'The test/scan shows that you/do not have X illness.'

Essentially, if the doctor says you have X psychiatric disorder, that is what you have. There is no proof, as other branches of medicine would understand it, and equally there is no disproof. If you disagree, you will find yourself simply in a battle of opinions in which the professional view trumps the lay one.

Second, and even more importantly, the problems that are called 'symptoms' in psychiatry are actually forms of thinking, feeling and behaving, not bodily complaints like pain or constant thirst or nausea. While these experiences may be unusual and upsetting – such as hearing hostile voices or having extreme mood swings – there are no universally agreed standards for deciding on 'normal' ways of feeling, thinking and behaving, because these judgements are subjective and depend on context. In fact, adding in the context often makes the experiences understandable. For example, the 'intense anger or difficulty controlling anger' that is said to be a 'symptom' of 'borderline personality disorder' may be an entirely reasonable response if you have been abused or abandoned, as many people with that label have. The experiences that are often diagnosed as 'depression' are known to arise more often when people are living in deprived areas and struggling to make ends meet. It is very strange logic to tell them they have coincidentally developed a 'mental illness' that needs treating with 'antidepressants' when their social circumstances give them so many reasons to be unhappy.

Interestingly, this reliance on subjective judgements rather than established biological signs is tacitly admitted within *DSM* itself in diagnostic criteria such as 'bizarre beliefs… that the person's culture would regard as totally implausible' and 'odd beliefs… inconsistent with cultural norms' (two of the supposed indications of 'schizophrenia'). This makes it clear that the criteria for making a psychiatric diagnosis are actually based on cultural standards about what is seen as acceptable in a particular society at a particular time. We would not introduce 'culture' into a legitimate medical diagnosis – either you have heart disease or a broken leg or you don't, wherever you live and whatever cultural group you belong to. But these criteria show that psychiatric diagnoses are ultimately based on social judgements, not medical ones. Some experiences, such as hearing voices, which are considered normal in some cultures, may be diagnosed even if they are a valued aspect of someone's life. These labels may well describe people with problems. They do not describe medical illnesses.

We are left with a process that is about as far from accepted scientific reasoning as you could get. In his revealing interviews with members of the *DSM* committees, James Davies reports one of them admitting:

> You must understand what I saw happening on these committees wasn't scientific – it more resembled a group of friends trying to decide where they want to go for dinner. One person says, 'I feel like Chinese food,' and another person says, 'No, no, I'm really more in the mood for Indian food,' and finally, after some discussion and collaborative give-and-take, they all decide to go have Italian. (Davies, 2013: 30)

In the meantime, the main defence of the current system is something along the lines of: 'We know that *DSM* is deeply flawed, but we have to stick with it until we come up with something better – although the necessary research will take years, possibly decades.' This seems to contradict another frank admission by Dr Allen Frances, chair of the *DSM-IV* committee: 'There is no definition of a mental disorder. I mean, you just can't define it. It's bullshit' (Greenberg, 2010).

For obvious reasons, it is very important that people who are diagnosed with 'bipolar disorder' or 'personality disorder' or 'depressive illness' or whatever are aware that this process has been described by the chair of the *DSM-IV* task force as 'bullshit'. We are simply being offered a circular pseudo-explanation of the kind: 'Why does this person hear hostile voices/have mood swings/feel suicidal?' 'Because they have psychosis/bipolar disorder/clinical depression.' 'How do you know they have psychosis/bipolar disorder/clinical depression?' 'Because they hear hostile voices/have mood swings/ feel suicidal.'

What are the implications?

If psychiatric diagnosis really doesn't have any sound basis in research, where does that leave psychiatry and the people who use its services? The implications call every aspect of current mental health practice into question – not just the labels and medical language but the over-reliance on drugs, the central role of doctors and nurses, the use of clinics and hospital settings rather than, say, crisis houses, therapy centres and advice bureaux, and so on. Almost every aspect of current practice and policy is based on the idea that extreme emotional distress is best understood as a kind of medical illness.

At this point, critics and supporters of the underlying medical model diverge, with supporters pinning their hopes on investing millions of dollars to develop replacement approaches that, they argue, will put diagnosis on a firmer, biologically based footing. Critics – many of whom come from within the psychiatric profession – believe that we have gone as far as we can down this particular road, and that 'It's time to reach beyond diagnostic dependence', in the words of psychiatrist Sami Timimi (2014). For example, the British Psychological Society (BPS) Division of Clinical Psychology issued a formal – and controversial – statement in 2013 calling for 'a paradigm shift in relation to the experiences that these diagnoses refer to, towards a conceptual system not based on a "disease" model'.

One absolutely clear implication of this situation is that service users and carers should be informed about these debates, rather than told that they have 'bipolar disorder' or 'personality disorder' or 'depressive illness', as if these were established facts. They should also be offered a genuine choice about whether they want to accept a psychiatric label. This doesn't mean that psychiatric drugs have no part to play, and nor does it mean refusing to support someone's benefit claims or withholding a label in any situation where it is currently necessary in order to access services. However, in my view, it does mean that it is no longer scientifically, professionally or ethically justifiable to insist on psychiatric diagnosis as the only way of describing people's distress and to deny people the opportunity to explore alternatives. Many of our most prominent mental health campaigners and activists have described how they took this step for themselves and, by doing so, eventually managed to free themselves from psychiatric services and a life in the role of 'psychiatric patient' (for examples, see Johnstone, 2014, Chapter 8).

In the meantime, it is important to be aware that it is perfectly possible to work with people in severe mental distress, including the more extreme forms we may refer to as 'psychosis', without using psychiatric diagnosis at all.

Formulation as an alternative to psychiatric diagnosis

Given the context described above, a range of alternatives to diagnosis has emerged, although they usually run alongside the traditional conceptualisations rather than replace them. They can perhaps be summarised as various ways of listening to people's stories – stories that are often obscured by a diagnosis and that very often involve trauma, abuse, loss, neglect, poverty and discrimination. Perhaps the most damaging aspect of psychiatric diagnosis is that it obscures these stories and their meanings.

One approach that is growing in popularity in mental health services is known as formulation. This can be described as an individual summary or story about the origins and meanings of a person's difficulties, which is developed jointly with them over a period of weeks or months. These personal narratives help to suggest interventions that are not based on the idea that the person is suffering from an 'illness' of some kind.

Here is an invented example:

> Karen was brought up by her mother, who suffered from depression. Her father left when she was three years old. Her mother remarried when Karen was seven. Her stepfather sexually abused her from age seven to 14.

> Karen was isolated and unhappy at school and started self-harming at age 11. She left school with few qualifications and had a series of relationships with men, some of which were abusive. She had a daughter with her husband, Steve. She left Steve because of his violence towards her, and is now single.

> When her daughter reached the age of seven, Karen's self-harming worsened and she became very desperate and low in mood.

Someone like Karen is at high risk of receiving one of the most stigmatising diagnoses, 'borderline personality disorder', with its damning message that you are not only mad but bad – fundamentally flawed in a way that is often assumed to be largely beyond treatment. In contrast to conditions like 'schizophrenia', a 'personality disorder' is not something you 'have' but something you 'are'.

And here is an alternative, a possible formulation, in which a client such as Karen and a professional, together, over a period of time, come up with a shared narrative based on two equally important forms of evidence: the professional's clinical experience and knowledge of the research, and the client's understanding of their own life and relationships and the sense they have made of them.

> Your early childhood experiences and relationships left you with very little sense of security or self-worth. Your father's departure felt like a major rejection and you saw yourself as unlovable and worthless. When your stepfather began to abuse you, his threats stopped you from telling anyone. Instead, you carried hidden feelings of guilt, anger and shame inside. Cutting yourself relieved these feelings when you couldn't express them in any other way. Desperate to find love and security, you often ended up with men who treated you badly. This confirmed your feelings of rejection and failure. You showed great courage in leaving your husband, and you very much want to give your daughter a better start in life. However, when she reached the age that your own abuse started, you could no longer push your feelings away. You felt overwhelmed with anger and distress and, with no one to support you, your self-harm became more frequent. Despite everything you have been through, you want to overcome your difficulties and use your strength and determination to build a different life for yourself and your daughter.

This shared hypothesis or 'best guess' about the origins of the client's distress can then become a guide to the intervention, while always being open to revision. Once you have a formulation that seems to offer a reasonable understanding of how the problems developed, an additional theory or hypothesis – such as, 'By the way, you are also feeling this way because you have a personality disorder/bipolar disorder/psychosis' – becomes entirely unnecessary. It is not an explanation; it adds nothing, and it undermines the formulation's positive message that distress can be understood in the context of someone's life.

Formulations, like anything else, can be carried out both helpfully and unhelpfully. Ideally, the client experiences a formulation as giving them a sense of understanding and hope; they feel they have been listened to and understood and that they have strengths and resources as well as difficulties. Guidelines setting out best practice in formulation have been published by the BPS Division of Clinical Psychology (DCP, 2011).

One of the helpful aspects of formulation is that it can offer a mid-point between the 'brain-or-blame' position that is so commonly seen in debates about diagnosis. We seem to find it hard to hold a middle ground between 'You have a physical illness, and therefore your distress is real and no one is to blame for it' and 'Your difficulties are imaginary and/or your or someone else's fault, and you ought to pull yourself together'. Given these apparently limited options, it is not surprising that many people choose to protect themselves against messages of blame and weakness by taking on a medical explanation, even if this means accepting the identity of being 'mentally ill', with all its consequences. Formulations, on the other hand, ideally convey the basic message: 'You are experiencing an understandable reaction to abnormal circumstances. Anyone else who had been through the same events might well have ended up feeling the same way.'

Team formulation

A variant of this process is known as team formulation, in which a whole mental health team comes together on a regular basis to develop a shared set of provisional ideas about a service user's difficulties. This can be seen as a kind of consultation or supervision process for the team. It needs to be done sensitively and collaboratively so that it feeds into a one-to-one formulation, and vice versa, with the service user's views being central. There is some evidence that team formulation can help staff to work cohesively together to support the service user and can minimise the risk of dismissive, blaming or rejecting messages from the staff (Johnstone & Dallos, 2014: Chapter 10).

The future of formulation

There has been a marked increase in the popularity of formulation, and several books on the subject have been published in recent years. However, while the growing tendency for all mental health professions to claim skills in formulation is welcome in one way, it may be concealing a less progressive agenda. In the face of growing criticism of diagnosis, some psychiatrists have started claiming that its flaws can be filled by formulation. As an editorial in the *British Journal of Psychiatry* puts it (Craddock & Mynors-Wallis, 2014):

> The key is to produce a formulation that… complements the diagnosis
> by including information about important clinical variables that have
> relevance for the management plan. We should continue to make diagnoses
> complemented by formulations.

But what the authors mean here is formulation as an addition, not an alternative, to diagnosis. It is the difference between describing someone as experiencing 'schizophrenia triggered by exam stress' and 'hearing the voice of your abuser due to unresolved feelings and memories' (see further below). The DCP guidelines (2011) describe this as the difference between *psychiatric* formulation and *psychological* formulation. This illustrates the constant danger that challenges to the psychiatric status quo will be stripped of their radical aspects and assimilated back into supporting the mainstream diagnostic model.

The trauma-informed approach

Formulation is one way of listening to people's stories. Another perspective on asking people about their experiences ('What happened to you?', not 'What's wrong with you?') is offered by the trauma-informed approach. This demonstrates that, as many of us have always known, the personal stories of people in mental distress are very often about various forms of trauma.

'Trauma' should be understood here in its wider sense, which includes emotional and physical abuse and neglect, domestic violence, bullying and many other adversities. The trauma-informed approach is based on a synthesis of findings from trauma studies, attachment theory and neuroscience, and integrates the causal roles of the mind, the body, relationships (particularly in early life) and the social world (for summaries, see Kezelman & Stavropoulos, 2012; van der Kolk, 2014). One such study is the now classic piece of research by Felitti and colleagues (1998), in which more than 17,000 members of the Kaiser Permanente insurance and healthcare provider in the US were asked whether they had experienced any of 10 forms of difficulty or household dysfunction in their early lives (so-called Adverse Childhood Experiences, or ACEs). These were:

- childhood maltreatment – sexual, verbal or physical abuse, emotional neglect, physical neglect
- household dysfunction – parent with diagnosis of 'mental illness', domestic violence, substance misuse, family member in prison, loss of a parent.

Subsequent research has expanded the list to include other adversities. This gives a score from 0 – for someone who experienced none of these events – to a possible 10 for someone who experienced all of them. A large and growing body of research has demonstrated that higher ACE scores are associated with a whole range of negative health, mental health, employment, educational and social outcomes. These include an increased risk of foetal death, injury and death in childhood, depression, suicide, 'psychosis', 'PTSD', drug use, criminal behaviour, heart disease, cancer, sexually transmitted diseases, lung disease, liver disease, smoking, obesity, diabetes, poor educational and work performance, homelessness, domestic violence, prostitution, unemployment and premature death.[1]

This should not be taken to mean that everyone who is bullied or abused will suffer long-term effects. Conversely, not everyone who seeks psychiatric help has

---

1. See www.acestoohigh.com (accessed 4 June 2019).

experienced obvious forms of trauma and deprivation. Research shows that there are a number of factors that, on average, make the long-term impact of adverse events more damaging, such as what age you were when the trauma occurred, how long it lasted, whether it was perpetrated by someone you depended on, and, perhaps most importantly, whether you had someone to confide in and protect you.

But each person's story is different, and a great deal will depend on the meaning the person attributes to their experiences. It is fairly obvious that someone who believes messages such as 'You are a bad little girl and if anyone finds out they will be angry' is likely to be left more distressed than someone who is encouraged to believe 'It was not your fault, it should never have happened to you, and you deserve to be protected.' Being heard, believed and having your experience validated by a friend, partner or professional can help to undo the damage and create new meanings that are to do with strength and survival.

We have known for years that traumas and adversities of various kinds are common in the lives of people who experience all forms of distress, from eating problems to 'borderline personality disorder', depression, anxiety, phobias and self-harm. This is also true for people diagnosed with 'schizophrenia' or 'psychosis'. For example, research indicates that people abused as children are 9.3 times more likely to develop 'psychosis', and for those suffering the severest kinds of abuse, the risk rises to 48 times (Janssen et al, 2004). People who have endured three kinds of abuse (eg. sexual, physical, bullying) are at an 18-fold higher risk of 'psychosis', and those experiencing five types are 193 times more likely to become 'psychotic' (Shevlin, Dorahy & Adamson, 2007). A recent large meta-analysis has established beyond any reasonable doubt that childhood adversity substantially increases the risk of the experiences we call 'psychosis' (Varese et al, 2012). The overall picture is irrefutable.

More recent research has focused not just on individual families and the specific events and circumstances described in the ACE studies but on people's wider environments too. When the ACE questions were repeated in inner-city Philadelphia, an area of high deprivation, the impact of environmental stressors such as racial discrimination or seeing someone being beaten, stabbed or shot emerged. These factors form the background to, and increase the likelihood of, abuse or neglect in relationships, and obviously have implications for wider social policy.[2]

From 'symptoms' to survival strategies

From a trauma-informed perspective, what the biomedical model calls 'symptoms' are not signs of illnesses to be 'treated' but survival strategies. Evidence from neuroscience shows that our minds and bodies have creative ways of coping

---

2. See www.philadelphiaaces.org/philadelphia-ace-survey (accessed 26 June 2019).

with emotionally overwhelming events and situations (see Chapter 5, Johnstone & Boyle, 2018a). We may go into an automatic fight/flight/freeze response to protect us from danger. We may cut off from feelings and memories that are too much to bear at the time, in a process called dissociation. For example, work by the Hearing Voices Network[3] has shown that hearing hostile and disturbing voices is often related to unresolved emotional trauma, and the voices may sound like or represent the person's abusers. All of these responses were essential at the time of the abuse but may become a problem in their own right if they continue once the threat has gone. The message of the trauma-informed approach is: 'You have survived very difficult circumstances in the best way you could at the time. These strategies are no longer needed or useful and, with the right kind of support, you can learn to leave them behind.'

Trauma-informed practice is based on a three-stage approach, as developed by Judith Herman (2001), although the stages may not be so clearly distinct from each other in practice. In Stage 1, education and stabilisation, people are introduced to the trauma-informed model and given information about the effects of adversity on the mind, brain and body. Once a degree of control and safety has been established, they may or may not wish to proceed to stage 2, trauma-processing work through various forms of therapy. In this stage, they are supported to revisit the traumatic memories and their associated meanings and feelings in order to resolve some of the emotional impact. Stage 3 is when people may be ready to move on in order to reconnect to their lives (Herman, 2001).

Although trauma-informed approaches originated in the US, they are gradually gaining influence in the UK. Population surveys of ACEs have been conducted in England, Wales and Scotland; the approach is recognised in official reports, and some services are adopting its ideas (Sweeney et al, 2018; see summary in Johnstone & Boyle, 2018a).

The Power Threat Meaning Framework

We have formulation as an alternative to diagnosis. We have the trauma-informed approach as an alternative to the biomedical model. Together, these encourage us to develop trauma-informed formulations as a basis for support with mental distress. A recent project draws on and expands both of these perspectives in order to suggest an overall framework that can move us beyond the medicalisation of distress once and for all.

The Power Threat Meaning Framework (PTMF), launched in January 2018, is an ambitious attempt to outline a conceptual alternative to the diagnostic model of psychological and emotional distress (Johnstone & Boyle, 2018a, 2018b).[4]

---

3. See www.intervoiceonline.org (accessed 4 June 2019).

4. The Power Threat Meaning Framework resources, videos and guided discussion can be found at www.bps.org.uk/news-and-policy/introducing-power-threat-meaning-framework (accessed 4 June 2019).

The PTMF was developed over a period of five years by a core group of clinical psychologists and former service users, supported by a range of other contributors, and was funded by the BPS Division of Clinical Psychology. In the relatively short time since its publication, it has attracted a great deal of interest within and beyond services, from service user groups, training courses, voluntary organisations, researchers and campaigners.[5]

The PTMF places formulation and trauma-informed practice within a much wider context of philosophical, psychological, sociological, political and therapeutic perspectives and approaches. It therefore uses the term 'narrative' to include not just formulation but any kind of meaning-making, whether inside or outside services, including art, music, poetry, community myths, rituals and ceremonies. Similarly, the PTMF places a strong emphasis on the socio-economic policies and contexts within which traumatic events arise, and on the largely unquestioned standards and ideals of Western industrialised societies that encourage us to feel shame and guilt if we are unable to live up to them. All of these can lead to distress, even if we have not experienced any of the commonly recognised 'traumas', as we struggle to find a sense of self-worth, meaning, identity and connection with others. Thus, the PTMF applies not just to people who have been diagnosed but to all of us.

A central aspect of the PTMF is its focus on the way power operates in our lives. It highlights the links between distress and social factors, such as poverty, discrimination, social exclusion and inequality, along with traumas such as abuse, neglect and violence. The role of ideological power – that is, the power to support certain interests through the language we use, the assumptions we make and the meanings we create – is less often recognised. However, ideological power is central to all other kinds of power. From a PTMF perspective, imposing a psychiatric label on someone is a very good example of the operation of this kind of power. As discussed above, these labels are not scientifically valid, and yet they often shape people's lives in very damaging ways. This is arguably in the interests of professionals, drug companies and, to an extent, society as a whole, as we are all shielded from looking too closely at the real root causes of distress.

The core PTMF questions

The PTMF integrates a great deal of evidence about the impact of these various forms of power in people's lives, the kinds of threat that misuses of power pose for us, and the ways we human beings have learned to respond to threat. In traditional mental health practice, these threat responses are sometimes called 'symptoms'.

The main aspects of the PTMF are summarised in these expanded versions of the core question, 'What has happened to you?'

---

5. See for example, *Clinical Psychology Forum* 2019; 313, January issue, for articles about the PTMF in practice. https://shop.bps.org.uk/publications/clinical-psychology-forum-no-313-january-2018.html (accessed 25 June 2019).

- 'What has happened to you?' (How is **power** operating in your life?)
- 'How did it affect you?' (What kind of **threats** does this pose?)
- 'What sense did you make of it?' (What is the **meaning** of these situations and experiences to you?)
- 'What did you have to do to survive?' (What kinds of **threat response** are you using?)

In addition, two further questions help us to think about what skills and resources individuals, families or social groups might have, and how we might pull all these ideas and responses together into a personal narrative or story:

- 'What are your strengths?' (What access to **power resources** do you have?)
- 'What is your story?' (How does all this fit together?)

These core questions can be used to help people to create more hopeful narratives or stories about their lives and the difficulties they may have faced or are still facing, instead of seeing themselves as blameworthy, weak, flawed or 'mentally ill'.[6]

General Patterns in distress

A central aspect of the PTMF is the attempt to outline patterns in the ways people respond to the negative impacts of power – in other words, to go beyond a series of individual narratives and identify broader regularities in people's expressions and experiences of distress.

From a PTMF viewpoint, the key difference between these 'General Patterns' and the patterns that support medical diagnosis are that they are *organised by meaning, not organised by biology*. They are fundamentally different from attempts to demonstrate, for example, that 'chemical imbalances cause depression'. Instead, the PTMF patterns are based on the evidence that people construct typical meanings in response to certain kinds of threat, such as feeling excluded, rejected, trapped, coerced or shamed, and may respond in characteristic ways. Thus, the patterns describe what people *do,* not illnesses they *have.* This is summarised in the phrase *patterns of embodied, meaning-based responses to threat.* It may be useful to draw on these patterns to help develop people's personal stories, and to convey a message of acceptance and validation, such as people sometimes find in diagnosis from knowing that they are not alone in their struggles.

If we return to Karen, whom we met earlier in the chapter, it is possible that she might feel her experiences are described by the General Pattern 'Surviving rejection, entrapment, and invalidation'. A short extract from this Pattern reads:

---

6. See Appendix 1, 'Guided Discussion', in Johnstone & Boyle, 2018b, for suggestions on how to apply these ideas and questions to your own life or that of someone you are working with.

> A central survival dilemma is maintaining attachments and relationships
> versus distrust and fear of rejection, hurt or harm… Sexual abuse is very
> common in the early lives of women who are described by this pattern.
> (Johnstone & Boyle, 2018b: 53)

It is important to note that the General Patterns go beyond typical formulations by making links to wider social and economic contexts, reducing the risk of self-stigma and self-blame by locating the roots of distress within wider socio-economic contexts. Thus, this Pattern also notes:

> These situations arise more frequently in power contexts of poverty, social
> inequality, unemployment, gender inequalities, and war… In service
> settings, the pattern is most frequently identified in women. This may result
> from the pathologising of responses such as anger or making demands
> that are seen as less acceptable in women. It may also relate to the fact that
> expressing anger inwardly, in line with female socialisation in some cultures,
> is more likely to result in a mental health referral than expressing anger
> outwardly in the form of violence to others. (Johnstone & Boyle, 2018b: 53)

In addition, the PTMF offers a new way of thinking about culturally specific understandings of distress. If patterns are based on meaning, not biology, we should not be surprised to find that experiences and expressions of distress are very different around the globe and in minority groups in the UK. The *DSM* response to this puzzling (from a medical viewpoint) fact is to try to translate these forms of distress back into the diagnostic model. The PTMF, on the other hand, encourages respect for the many creative and non-medical ways of understanding distress around the world, and the varied forms of narrative and healing practices that may be used.

This overarching framework is not intended to replace all the ways we currently think about and work with distress. Instead, the aim is to support and strengthen the many examples of good practice that already exist, while also suggesting new ways forward. These may or may not include standard interventions such as psychiatric drugs or therapy, but there is an equally strong emphasis on the need to look at the wider circumstances of social injustice and inequality in people's lives, to restore the links between personal distress and social injustice, and to take action at that level as well. The PTMF takes us beyond the individual and shows that we are all part of a wider struggle for a fairer society.

Summary

As I have argued, the alternative to diagnosis is listening to people's stories. These stories may be about trauma or abuse in their most recognisable forms. They may be about the more subtle but corrosive impacts of poverty, discrimination, exclusion and marginalisation. They may take the form of perceived failure to live up to societal expectations. Or they may well be a mixture of all of these. Everyone's story is unique and, at the same time, everyone's story is rooted in our shared struggle to survive and find meaning and connection in an increasingly individualistic, materialistic, fragmented, unequal and unjust society.

In her classic book, *Trauma and Recovery*, Judith Herman captures the flavour of the stories behind the labels:

> The knowledge of horrible events periodically intrudes into public awareness but is rarely retained for long… Clinicians know the privileged moment of insight when repressed ideas, feelings, and memories surface into consciousness… Victims who have been silenced begin to reveal their secrets… Survivors challenge us to reconnect fragments, to reconstruct history, to make meaning of their present symptoms in the light of past events. (Herman, 2001: 2)

The chapters in this book are a contribution to that process.

References

American Psychiatric Association (2013). *Diagnostic and Statistical Manual of Mental Disorders* (5th ed) (*DSM-5*). Washington, DC: APA.

Craddock N, Mynors-Wallis L (2014). Psychiatric diagnosis: impersonal, imperfect and important. *The British Journal of Psychiatry 204*(2): 93-95.

Cromby J, Harper D, Reavey P (eds) (2013). *Psychology, Mental Health and Distress*. Basingstoke: Palgrave Macmillan.

Davies J (2013). *Cracked: why psychiatry is doing more harm than good*. London: Icon Books.

Division of Clinical Psychology (2013). *Classification of Behaviour and Experience in Relation to Functional Psychiatric Diagnosis: time for a paradigm shift*. Leicester: British Psychological Society.

Division of Clinical Psychology (2011). *Good Practice Guidelines on the Use of Psychological Formulation*. Leicester: British Psychological Society.

Felitti V, Anda R, Nordenberg D, Williamson DF, Spitz AM, Edwards V Koss MP, Marks JS (1998). Relationship of childhood abuse and household dysfunction to many of the leading causes of death in adults: the Adverse Childhood Experiences (ACE) study. *American Journal of Preventive Medicine 14*(4): 245–258.

Frances A (2013). *Saving Normal: an insider's revolt against out-of-control psychiatric diagnosis, DSM-5, big pharma, and the medicalization of ordinary life*. New York, NY: Harper Collins.

Greenberg G (2010). Inside the battle to define mental illness. [Online.] *Wired*; 27 December. www.wired.com/magazine/2010/12/ff_dsmv/ (accessed 25 June 2019).

Herman JL (2001). *Trauma and Recovery: the aftermath of violence – from domestic abuse to political terror*. New York, NY: Basic Books.

Janssen I, Krabbendam L, Bak M, Hanssen M, Vollebergh W, de Graaf R, van Os J (2004). Childhood abuse as a risk factor for psychotic experiences. *Acta Psychiatrica Scandinavica 109*: 38–45.

Johnstone L (2018). Madness and the family – the re-emergence of Laingian ideas. *Journal of Psychosocial Studies 11*(2): 32–49.

Johnstone L (2014). *A Straight Talking Introduction to Psychiatric Diagnosis*. Ross-on-Wye: PCCS Books.

Johnstone L, Boyle M, with Cromby J, Dillon J, Harper D, Kinderman P, Longden E, Pilgrim D, Read J (2018a). *The Power Threat Meaning Framework: towards the identification of patterns in emotional distress, unusual experiences and troubled or troubling behaviour, as an alternative to functional psychiatric diagnosis*. Leicester: British Psychological Society.

Johnstone L, Boyle M, with Cromby J, Dillon J, Harper D, Kinderman P, Longden E, Pilgrim D, Read J (2018b). *The Power Threat Meaning Framework: overview*. Leicester: British Psychological Society.

Johnstone L, Dallos R (eds) (2014). *Formulation in Psychology and Psychotherapy: making sense of people's problems* (2nd ed). London: Routledge.

Kezelman CA, Stavropoulos PA (2012). *Practice Guidelines for Treatment of Complex Trauma and Trauma-Informed Care and Service Delivery*. Milsons Point: Blue Knot Foundation. www.blueknot.org.au (accessed 10 June 2019).

Pies R (2014). Nuances, narratives and the chemical imbalance theory in psychiatry. [Online.] *Medscape*; 15 April. www.medscape.com/viewarticle/823368 (accessed 24 June 2019).

Read J, Dillon J (eds) (2013). *Models of Madness: psychological, social and biological approaches to psychosis* (2nd ed). London: Routledge (pp191–209).

Read J, Sanders P (2010). *A Straight Talking Introduction to the Causes of Mental Health Problems*. Ross-on-Wye: PCCS Books.

Shevlin M, Dorahy M, Adamson G (2007). Trauma and psychosis: an analysis of the National Comorbidity Survey. *American Journal of Psychiatry 164*(1): 166–169.

Sweeney A, Filson B, Kennedy A, Collinson S, Gillard S (2018). A paradigm shift: relationships in trauma-informed mental health services. *BJP Advances 24*: 319–333.

Timimi S (2014). First do no harm. *Clinical Psychology Forum 261*: 6–8.

van der Kolk B (2014). *The Body Keeps the Score: brain, mind, and body in the healing of trauma*. London: Allen Lane.

Varese F, Smeets F, Drukker M, Ritsaert L, Lataster T, Viechtbauer W (2012). Childhood adversities increase the risk of psychosis. *Schizophrenia Bulletin 38*: 661–671.

World Health Organization (2018). *International Classification of Diseases* (11th review). Geneva: World Health Organization.

2 | Counselling, psychotherapy, diagnosis and the medicalisation of distress

Pete Sanders

'Colin Baker, for Thames News, Westminster... soaked, with cold feet and an aching heart... pissed off, really dreadfully pissed off.'[1]

Psychodiagnosis[2] is a contentious subject and practice. If it were not, there would be no need for this book, or for the mountain of critical literature, research and data analysis that it is part of and the countless groups – including Drop the Disorder! – convened explicitly to challenge it. Everyone would welcome their *psycho*diagnosis, as we do when our GP tells us there is a name for the physical pain we are suffering that not only explains it but identifies its cure. But hundreds of thousands of people worldwide refer to themselves as victims or survivors of a medicalised system driven by psychodiagnosis, so all is not well.

It is one of the lynchpins of medicalisation – a scientific approach to human suffering based on positivism and experimental method. We are socialised into a world where an increasing number of daily activities and everyday experiences are medicalised. That is, they are spoken about in terms of what is normal and abnormal, with the outer reaches of abnormality being pathological – that is, a 'disorder' or 'illness'. This phenomenon is creeping over our entire lives, insinuating itself into every nook and cranny of our public and private selves.

---

1. See www.youtube.com/watch?v=EVYhCBVKfW8 (accessed 25 June 2019).

2. I am using this term because 'diagnosis' in normal use has too broad a meaning and automatically includes the sense in which it is used to mean the discernment of physical illnesses.

Two types of psychodiagnosis

There are at least two types or levels of psychodiagnosis. First is what we might call 'psychiatric psychodiagnosis', where a person's signs and symptoms are scrutinised and an 'illness' or 'disorder' is identified by their unique pattern. In physical medicine, this makes sense and, more importantly, is backed up by demonstrable cause-and-effect relationships.

Second is the theory and practice of micro-psychodiagnosis, which I will call 'intervention diagnosis'. This diagnosis takes place inside or between the therapy sessions and is done by therapists who practise as experts with professional skills in a model that hypothesises that the therapists have access to special knowledge unavailable to the person in distress. On the basis of this moment-to-moment diagnosis, the psychological practitioner selects interventions, based on theory, training, clinical experience, personal preferences, hunches and idiosyncratic taxonomies of behaviours and experiences, also known as 'signs' and 'symptoms'.[3]

In the literature, we find a range of different viewpoints, from outright supporters to outright critics, and it is increasingly popular to say psychodiagnosis requires 'nuanced' examination. Some commentators, theorists and practitioners would have it that the first type, psychiatric diagnosis, lacks evidence and is invalid and unreliable, while intervention diagnosis is fine and necessary to practise integrated, pluralistic or even 'client-centred' therapies. These descriptions and arguments are not new; indeed, it may surprise some to know that they once represented the status quo in counselling, if not psychotherapy, in the UK. How and why practice has changed is a matter of opinion, and I will suggest a couple of explanations along the way. In this chapter, I represent the counsellors and psychotherapists who say psychodiagnosis is just wrong, plain and simple, from top to bottom, whichever way you look at it, psychiatric or interventional. I will look critically at the place of diagnosis in counselling and psychotherapy[4] (spoiler alert: there is no place for it), while pondering why the counselling and psychotherapy profession steadfastly keeps its mouth shut when the topic of the medicalisation of distress comes up. Craig Newnes (1999) noted that it is power struggles between competing moral, political and economic authorities, rather than science, that have determined who is responsible for the wellbeing of our mental life.

---

3. I use the term 'experiences' throughout unless specifically writing about the medical model, since 'symptoms' is a medical term and its use accepts the contested assumption that we are dealing with illnesses, rather than the diversity of human experience (a phenomenological, psychotherapeutic view). I briefly state my position regarding language later in this chapter and Clare Shaw writes about it in Chapter 7.

4. I do not think there is any difference between the practice of counselling and psychotherapy – save cash, power and ego-riddled turf wars – except that counselling is mercifully theory-lite (when relieved of the burden of diagnosis). Therefore, I ungrammatically refer to counselling and psychotherapy as a singular entity.

Today, in the 21st century, we are faced with a complex, multi-faceted system, the characteristics of which include being, among other things, a system for healing; a scientific enterprise; a means of employment for psychologists, psychiatrists and associated trades; a professional hierarchy where reputations can be made and broken; a state-control mechanism; a sanctuary to escape the overwhelm of disintegrating social relations in daily life, and an adjunct to the pharmaceutical industry (adapted from Newnes, 1999: 22).

Psychiatric psychodiagnosis

Psychiatric psychodiagnosis occupies a peculiar position of simultaneous strength *and* vulnerability in both Western culture in general and in counselling and psychotherapy. On the one hand, it is the lynchpin of the culturally endorsed medical model of mental illness and the medicalisation of distress, seemingly fulfilling a need to believe that, if we name something, we have power over it. The *DSM-5* and *ICD-11* psychiatric psychodiagnostic manuals, published by the American Psychiatric Association (2013) and the World Health Organization (2018) respectively, claim to be taxonomies of illnesses, backed by science. On the other hand, there is substantial – some would say overwhelming – evidence that these psychodiagnostic systems are flawed and unscientific – both invalid and unreliable,[5] as valid and reliable as astronomy:

> Like star signs, diagnoses fail on all of these counts, and peddle meaningless generalisations ('schizophrenia is the result of an interaction between genes and the environment') or extravagant but unsubstantiated claims ('schizophrenia is a disease of the dopamine system') as if they are scientific truths. (Bentall, 2004: 194)

They are nothing more than useless taxonomies of experiences,[6] with the aim of medicalising everyday life and medicating diversity for profit and control.[7]

Intervention diagnosis

There are many ways in which theory translates into practice in counselling. One is the degree to which the approach has a theory with a taxonomy embedded within it – that is, a way of categorising client experiences or behaviours, types of interventions and how an intervention might fit, or be an appropriately tailored (ie. therapeutic) response to, a type of behaviour or experience. Some therapeutic approaches have elaborate systems of such micro-diagnoses of client behaviour

---

5. A rather damning indictment since their only substantial claim is to represent science and the triumph of our 'understanding' of the mind-body connection.

6. See footnote 2 p.24.

7. Some insist on a more nuanced argument, looking at how experiences cluster.

in order to determine the 'correct' therapeutic response. This whole process is almost always hidden from the client, and this mystery confers on the therapist the authority of the appearance of *knowledge* of the (hidden) lexicon and method of the system, from which the client is excluded. Even the appearance of knowledge, in the medicalised psychodiagnostic psychotherapy interview, is power.

Later in this chapter I mention what Orne (1962) called the 'demand characteristics' of the situation – namely, a person's tendency to conform to what they think are the expected outcomes of a given situation. Draw your own conclusions about what is expected of a client when the therapist acts as though they are channelling some greater source of scientific knowledge. The antidote to this is that, while clients might be extremely upset and distressed, they are not stupid. They respond to the demand characteristics of a counselling interview in a number of ways, depending on the urgency and level of distress they are experiencing, but wherever possible turn the therapeutic relationship, and their understanding of it, to their own understanding of healing. Bohart and Tallman (1999, 2010) detail how clients creatively interpret even crass mistakes by the therapist in their effort to heal themselves.

Diagnosis and medicalisation in counselling and psychotherapy practice

The importance of how we talk

The importance of language in the realm of unusual and/or distressing experiences cannot be overstated, because language is able to both *describe* and potentially *determine* human experience. Regardless of the old saying 'Sticks and stones may break my bones, but names will never hurt me', bullying, stigmatisation and discrimination all have their foundations in name-calling and violent language, causing significant distress. Language can and does *hurt* via stigmatisation, and it happens to people on the receiving end of a socially difficult or simply unwelcome psychiatric diagnostic label. The acknowledgement of the severity of this additional distress has led to a series of anti-stigmatisation initiatives. Unfortunately, all concern themselves with educating the general public as to the 'facts' about 'mental illness' – none of them advocate the obvious: simply putting an end to psychiatric psychodiagnosis and medicalisation.

In addition to its capacity to hurt and exclude people (even accidentally), we know that language can support, heal, uplift and inspire us as well. In fact, helping in counselling depends upon a real connection and communication (using language or otherwise) between the counsellor and client in which 1) the client is able to describe their sense of hurt and the difficulties they experience in their world, and 2) the counsellor consciously uses the spoken word[8] to communicate

---

8. Readers can use their imagination to translate these ideas into non-verbal therapy modalities – art, music, dance, movement.

understanding, comfort and desire for healing. The common powerful message from many practitioners is that, when communicating with people in distress, it is imperative to use the same types of words, the same vocabulary that they use to describe their experiences. We need to understand, as best we are able, what it is like to live in their world, as if we were them.

For a number of well-documented reasons, like it or not, therapists are voices of authority in society and in individual helping relationships (Proctor, 2018), which means that what we say counts. People take notice when a newspaper or news bulletin declares, 'A psychologist says …', and, in their worst moments of despair, people listen for the slightest hints of advice and words of direction from their therapist, regardless of what idiosyncratic nonsense we are spouting and even in the absence of the therapist saying anything at all.[9] These dynamics, well known to psychologists but hardly allowed for in our understanding of power in therapy, are called the 'demand characteristics' of the situation (Orne, 1962). Look it up – it's free online… you'll not know whether to laugh or cry. It is easy to adjust Orne's words to substitute a therapy situation for his original psychology experiment situation. Then, after Orne (1962: 777), we might say that therapy is a special form of social interaction. The client places themselves under the control of the therapist and may agree to tolerate a considerable degree of discomfort, boredom or actual pain, if required to do so.

The situation is made worse if the therapist is entrenched in the medical model, with its established, comforting role power, and uses diagnosis-speak with exotic terms that appear to reinforce the specious expert status of the speaker. Therapists are influencers. If we talk sick, our clients will – beyond their own already confusing and frightening experiences – think sick or have it confirmed that they are sick, and are more likely to feel sick and act sick. Is it good practice for counsellors and psychotherapists to use psychiatric psychodiagnoses with their clients when there is no evidence that they actually exist as disease entities, yet there *is* evidence that the resulting stigmatisation causes further distress?

It is a short step from support of *psychiatric* psychodiagnosis and the utility of categorisation *per se* to the use of intervention diagnosis. Many models, from transactional analysis (eg. Ware, 1983), through CBT to contemporary psychoanalysis and, for example, mentalization (eg. Bateman & Fonagy, 2016), incorporate systems of categorisation (aka diagnosis) into their theory and practice. Indeed, it is a mark of best practice to be able to quickly and confidently[10]

---

9. Therapists give dodgy advice all the time, but more often than not when they feel completely stumped and the client seems most overtly distressed and stuck. Listening and accompanying someone in the middle range of experiences is easy.

10. Of course, speed and particularly 'confidence' are the least important, effective and relationship-orientated 'skills' required for decent psychotherapy. They operate from outside the other person's frame of reference, work against collaboration and exude signals of the therapist's adroit cleverness and power. Decent psychotherapy demands humility, tentativeness and permission-seeking at a pace that suits building and maintaining a safe relationship. Nothing more, nothing less.

categorise a person by their behaviour and/or their description of their experiences and select an appropriate therapeutic response. The problem with these methods is that they all make an external expert judgement on a person's experiences, with a view to advising on a recommended change process. The process goes as follows:

1. Observe patient from the frame of reference of the theory.
2. Identify pathological behaviours and/or experiences as per theory.
3. Select corrective interventions from theory.
4. Apply corrective interventions.
5. Assess result using diagnostic process from (1).

This is the identical procedure followed by a medical practitioner in a medical model using psychiatric psychodiagnosis. It is predicated on the assumed expertise of the psychological practitioner – an expertise that has little more validity and reliability than the *DSM-5* and *ICD-11* and their associated treatments. With increasing numbers of counsellors and psychotherapists completing doctorates of one sort or another, the illusion of medical expertise is enhanced. The practitioner is further removed from the position of collaborator and companion, which a few years ago was the favoured, indeed essential, character of the counsellor.

One defence of these in-therapy, moment-to-moment micro-diagnoses is that they are more closely informed by the distressed person's experiences and led by empathy, or interest, in the person's narrative, in their story. Such explanations are fanciful, since both psychiatric psychodiagnosis and micro-intervention diagnosis are led not by empathy for empathy's sake but by the drive to fit the client and their behaviour and experiences into a model. This is the use of empathy as a tool, for the sake of the implicit therapeutic power of being received and understood, not holding an attitude of empathic acceptance for its own sake (see Grant, 1990).

The importance of how we listen

Dispensing with intervention diagnosis would be unpopular for a number of reasons. It shows us that counsellors and psychotherapists are not experts – they have no better understanding of distress than the general public (clients) in the sense that there is no single theory of types of behaviour or clusters of experiences that explains your, my or anyone's particular distress. Therefore, there cannot be a list of therapeutic techniques that ties in neatly. Saying that it is complex and requires a complex theory is not right either. It just adds to the growing telephone directory of new theories, arguments, debates and 'evidence' and old theories renamed and recycled. Our experience shows that everyone's distress is different, and no theory of categories can cope with that, since there are just as many categories as there are people. When counsellors and psychotherapists say that everyone is unique, it should not be a trite cliché. It must be a banner of truth under which people in distress and psychological practitioners can gather, knowing that all stories of fear, darkness, pain and joy will be heard patiently, fully and without judgement.

Here lies the actual expertise of a counsellor and psychotherapist. Although such listening can come naturally to a few people, most of us need to learn (or re-learn) how to listen this way. The learning is nothing to do with personality types, lists of symptoms or pathological behaviours, since they, along with our own ideas and predilections for 'sane' behaviour, are at best distractions that get in the way. No structure is imposed in this way of listening; rather, it involves simply being with the other person and helping them struggle towards their own understanding. This means that they make their own meaning for their experiences, invent their own theory for healing, try it out, and occasionally fail along the way. That is why a good deal of decent therapy is called support.

The skill is to be able to get out of the way while still being present for the person. But this is more difficult than it seems. It is possible to get too far out of the way and appear distant or not present. Equally, we might think we are getting out of the way but our own ideas just creep in. Perhaps we have helped ourselves or someone else before in a particular way and we just can't shift that old method that was such a success. Perhaps we are frightened or upset by what the person is telling us. Perhaps we are worried that they are not feeling any better or they seem to be getting worse. The way to deal with all of these interferences and distractions is *not* to interrogate the person we are trying to help more closely, or make suggestions, or read about other distressed people's experiences, or check that they are being completely forthright. The helper must ask *themselves* what they are doing or not doing that might be getting in the way. Scott D Miller and colleagues (2016) suggest a simple solution: ask the client how you're doing and what, if anything, they are finding helpful. Hardly any kind of science at all really; certainly not rocket science.

Those in favour of the demedicalisation of distress

Readers will have realised that I am not challenging diagnosis and medicalisation with a balanced, evidence-based argument. As I have already made clear, this chapter does not present 'both sides'. We live in a world where psychodiagnosis is assumed to be logical, scientifically sensible, necessary and truthful. This is the air we breathe and its over-representation in the professional and general culture needs no further platform here. Any dissenting voices and criticisms of diagnosis and the medicalisation of distress are labelled as unevidenced, subjective, politically motivated, rhetorical, and therefore irresponsible, as they appeal to, and hold out false hope to, impressionable, vulnerable people. The rhetoric of the privileged dominant medical establishment further constructs critical voices as sounding unnecessarily loud or angry. There is not time or space to challenge much of this in this chapter, and other chapters in this book do it better. Nevertheless, it is worth considering Guy Debord's words:

> This… should be read bearing in mind that it was written with the deliberate intention of doing harm to spectacular society. There was never anything outrageous, however, about what it had to say. (Debord, 1994)

Traditional psychological care remains 'a vast human experiment' (Newnes, 1999: 22) and comes with the following attributes, which are easily identified and, where necessary, destroyed with scientific, moral and lived-experience ordinance in any critical response:

1. It medicalises distress.
2. It is reductionistic and symptom orientated and reproduces an unevidenced psychopathology.
3. The service provider is constructed as a professional, technician and expert.
4. The person cared for is constructed as a patient, ill, broken or deficient.
5. The problem is constructed as imbalance, deficiency or illness.
6. The power relations between the professional and the person cared for are complex, largely unacknowledged and predisposed to compliance and coercion.
7. The power relations are acted out in the form of 'treatment'. Commonly offered models are instructional and correctional, reinforcing both a deficiency and illness model and the low structural and personal power of the patient.
8. The change process is constructed as an administered correctional treatment technology featuring repair or reprogramming.
9. The aim of treatment is to recover a previous state of being, correct deviance and return the patient to their social and occupational milieus.
10. It is unevidenced, and its apparatus (eg. diagnostic categories) is unreliable and invalid.

This system of understanding also represents the assertion, in the name of science, of a triumph of technology over nature in the domain of counselling and psychotherapy. It values:

- outcome over process – 'ends' rather than 'means'
- objectivity over subjectivity
- reductionism – atomisation of human personhood and experience
- analysis over synthesis – human beings seen as machines rather than complex dynamical systems

- the abstraction of facts over the description of experiences – more subjugation of humans as holistic beings in favour of humans as machines
- people as objects over people as persons.

Together and individually this list is the antithesis of counselling and psychotherapy. In 1976, when interviewed by psychiatrist Anthony Clare for the BBC Radio programme *All in the Mind*, Carl Rogers said:

> We regard the medical model as an extremely inappropriate model for dealing with psychological disturbances. The model that makes more sense is a growth model or a developmental model. In other words, we see people as having a potential for growth and development, and that that can be released under the right psychological climate. We don't see them as sick and needing a diagnosis, prescription and a cure. And that is a very fundamental difference with a good many implications. (Rogers, 1976)

Rogers' words, like so much of person-centred psychology, tend to be dismissed as irrelevant, out of date or otherwise not fit for the 21st century. It is interesting, then, that the key elements of his historic operationalisation of the helping relationship (empathy, non-judgemental respect and genuineness) continue to this day to be re-invented by adherents of other approaches. You've probably read about them, with their new names and new acronyms, but it's the same old Rogerian wine in new, fancy, expensive bottles.

Another key contribution made in 1976, ignored by the profession of counselling and psychotherapy, is the short monograph *Medical Nemesis* by Ivan Illich. In it he describes three levels of *iatrogenesis*, or harm caused by structures and activities intended to cure, that result from the false diagnosis of 'non-diseases' and the over-activity and over-confidence of the medical establishment. These are:

- clinical iatrogenesis – the harm done to patients by medical treatments
- social iatrogenesis – the damage done by the unnecessary medicalisation of life (which he called polyphragmasia), and
- cultural iatrogenesis – the destruction of culturally traditional ways of dealing with pain, illness and death.

The medicalisation of distress results in all three levels of damage: clinical, social and cultural. It insinuates clinical methods, supported by social structures, and reproduces cultural milieus that are technological, objective, atomised and reductionistic, treatment- and dosage-oriented, commodified and consumerised. Illness metaphors have become woven into the fabric of cultural responses to practically all of our ordinary, natural, *everyday* life events: birth, childhood and child-rearing, adolescence, relationship breakdown, family disturbance, emotional pain, death and grief… the list goes on. The medical model wrestled with religion and local cultural rituals for control of these events and won. In 2019 we find cardiologists meeting with government ministers to tackle over-diagnosis and over-treatment with statins while the helping professions invent new therapies for new psychological disorders every day. Our professional journals are bulging, and it seems that there really is no end to the new ways we can become mentally ill. Nikolas Rose's (1985) Psy Complex is thriving.

A historical excursion: psychotherapy imitating medicine

Medical historians tracing the evolution of European medicine as philosophy, theory and practice note that medicine started as a *biographical* or *bedside* activity. Physicians didn't have science to guide their actions. At best, they implied an authoritative pseudoscience in the presence of patients. This promoted the use of leeches, poisons, fasting, diets, fresh air and an almost endless list of patented treatments. Brennan and Hollanders (2004) state that, during this early stage, 'the power balance between practitioner and patient was relatively equal and the approach idiosyncratic, determined by the preference and worldview of the patient'.

Next came the stage where practitioners established a standardised, scientific, medical approach. This promoted a new range of poisons, diets and physical interventions permitted by advances in pharmacology and technology. During this stage, as doctors became more expert, 'patients became more passive and lacking in individuality' (Brennan & Hollanders, 2004: 123). The current stage is epitomised by medical reductionism concerned with microscopic causes of disease: genetics and neurobiology. It is a model of laboratory medicine, with associated biotechnical and pharmaceutical industries, the patient relegated to being the envelope, carrier or conduit through which such medicine can be practised. Their humanity is an unnecessary and often unwelcome obstruction.

There are striking parallels with the profession of counselling and psychotherapy. When I trained as a counsellor in 1974, there was no 'profession' of counselling, just a handful of one-year, full-time counselling courses at postgraduate level. Most courses were person-centred with a bit of what would now be considered to be 'old-fashioned' behaviour therapy using operant and classical conditioning.

These were the days when counsellors offered unlimited sessions, generic practice and a 'bedside' (literally, in the case of counselling people with AIDS, for example) practice. Private practice in counselling was practically unheard of and those who weren't working in education or for statutory services were volunteers with, for example, the National Marriage Guidance Council (now Relate).

Now, further mimicking medicine, practice has to be evidence-based and we are overseen by a clinical regulatory body, the National Institute for Health and Care Excellence (NICE). Any decent 1970s psychologist would challenge the faux-medical randomised controlled trial methodology and the mountains of poor, unreplicated, small-sample research now being presented for review. Furthermore, the media, with its populist portrayals of science, have rendered us unable to tell the difference between fact and fiction. Counsellors and psychotherapists the world over are trying desperately to show how grown up they are by mentioning either neuroscience or psychogenetics.

Differences between medicalised and non-medicalised helping

So, what are the characteristics of the offer of counselling and psychotherapy? What are the differences between a counselling model of distressing experience and a medicalised model of distress? I made my best effort at summarising this 14 years ago (Sanders, 2005: 23), after the work of Blackburn and Yates (2004) on models of learning disability, and have since developed it, as follows.

Table 1: Differences between medicalised and non-medicalised helping

	Counselling (humanistic/person-centred/non-diagnostic)	Medicalised, diagnostic and instrumental models
Metaphors for distress	Self-defined, described experience of distress Actualisation/natural response to trauma Diversity Changeable	Sick, ill, damaged Imbalance Exogenous treatment Disability Immutable
Vocabulary	Potentiality and diversity	Deficiency and normalisation
Authority	Client	Therapist
Privileged professional discourse	Nothing above service user/client's experience	Anyone except the service user/client (in order of power) Psychiatrist Clinical psychologist/psychotherapist Psychiatric nurse/social worker

Power relations between client and practitioner	Acknowledged Informed by dynamics of person being helped as self-directing healer Reinforces personal power of person being helped	Where acknowledged, informed by need for treatment compliance, therefore predisposed to abuse Reinforces low structural and personal power of patient
Nature and process of intervention	Holistic, integrated Respectful of client autonomy – emphasises and strengthens personal power of client Empathy, description Celebrates potentiality and diversity, uniqueness Accompaniment	Reductionistic, atomistic Diagnosis Instructional Correctional Reinforces deficiency model Prescription
Nature of distressed person	Whole person Client Director of healing process Represented by experience	Compartmentalised Patient Deficient Represented by taxonomy of symptoms
Nature of therapist	Companion, collaborator	Expert, professional, technician, physician
Privileged frame of reference	Internal (person-being helped)	External (theory, system, helper)
Change process	Self-directed Growth Actualisation Insight Development	Insight Repair Extinction/relearning Reprogramming Cure

Aim of intervention	Fulfilment of potential Celebration of personhood and diversity	Recover previous state of being (health) Return to homoeostatic balance
Resources	In a rich, facilitative, growth-orientated milieu the client is able to make use of all possible resources, including the whole person of client	Expertise of therapist Psychopharmacology Psychotechnology

This comparison is not simply between a medical model and a counselling model of psychological helping. It is also between the past and the present in counselling and psychotherapy, as profession and practice increasingly mimic medicine.

The challenge for counselling and psychotherapy

This chapter is a mash up of things I have been saying and writing for more than 30 years. At various points over those years, I believed that things had changed. But no. Groups like Drop the Disorder! are a continuing reminder that much work still needs to be done. In this world of increasing professionalisation at any cost, service users and practitioners (the same group, since we all might need help for distress at any time) are living with the price paid.

How should the profession respond? I can do no better than paraphrase something I wrote with Keith Tudor nearly 20 years ago (Sanders & Tudor, 2001: 157). In our 'manifesto', as we called it – a prescription as yet unfulfilled – we suggested that counsellors and psychotherapists:

- base their practice on a thorough and critical understanding of psychiatry and psychotherapy *in context*…
- strive to facilitate the reclaiming by clients of personal power in therapeutic relationships characterised by collaborative power…
- reflect in their practice the awareness that the struggle for mental health involves changing society…
- organise and challenge oppressive institutions, especially psychiatric hegemony in the organisation of mental health services, professional monopoly on the control of service provision and direction, and the colonisation of the voluntary sector in mental health…
- support the service-user movement in general and, in particular, service-user involvement in mental health service development and service user-controlled alternatives to psychiatric services…

- remain open to alternatives (eg. as regards 'treatment') and seek to build alliances that emphasise user/survivor perspectives (on, among other issues, hearing voices and survivor-controlled alternatives), and encourage and promote greater public access to information through new technology as challenging the knowledge-based power of professionals.

While clinical psychologists have stood alongside survivors/users of mental health services to mount a sustained critique of medicalisation and diagnosis, counsellors and psychotherapists have been notable by their absence. There is a similar absence of critical publications in counselling and psychotherapy. Despite widespread discrediting and rejection of *DSM-5*, from its bereavement exclusion[11] to its descriptions of personality disorder, the profession of counselling and psychotherapy remains in thrall to psychodiagnosis. Indeed, in the continued absence of any evidence that distress should be thought of as an *illness*, medicalisation actually continues to gain ground; new disorders are announced every year, with hardly a word of protest from counselling and psychotherapy professional bodies or their members. Could it be that the whole profession is pleased that broadening the range of diagnoses might result in an increase in footfall? Is that the problem?

Binding the profession to psychodiagnosis is unscientific and unethical, and will come unstuck. Professional bodies should act now with integrity to lead therapists and public alike towards a non-medicalised understanding of human distress.

Pete Sanders, my views are my own, Mid-Wales, tired, old, with a dodgy and aching heart, still waiting for change… pissed off, really dreadfully pissed off.

References

American Psychiatric Association (2013). *Diagnostic and Statistical Manual of Mental Disorders* (5th ed). Washington, DC: APA.

Bateman A, Fonagy P (2016). *Mentalization-Based Treatment for Personality Disorders: a practical guide.* Oxford: Oxford University Press.

---

11. The 'bereavement exclusion' was a clause in *DSM-IV* stating that a person experiencing grief following the death of a close relative or friend should not be diagnosed with 'Major Depressive Disorder' (MDD) on the grounds that symptoms would likely be caused by a normal process of grief. In *DSM-5*, this exclusion was removed, meaning that a diagnosis of MDD could be given if 'symptoms' persist two weeks after bereavement, thus medicalising grief.

Bentall RP (2004). Abandoning the concept of schizophrenia: the cognitive psychology of hallucinations and delusions. In: Read J, Mosher LR, Bentall RP (eds). *Models of Madness: psychological, social and biological approaches to schizophrenia.* Hove: Brunner-Routledge (pp195–208).

Blackburn P, Yates C (2004). Same story – different tale. *Mental Health Today December:* 31–33.

Bohart AC, Tallman K (2010). Clients as active self-healers: implications for the person-centered approach. In: Cooper M, Watson JC, Hölldampf D (eds). *Person-Centred and Experiential Therapies Work: a review of the research on counselling, psychotherapy and related practices.* Ross-on-Wye: PCCS Books.

Bohart AC, Tallman K (1999). *How Clients Make Therapy Work: the process of active self-healing.* Washington, DC: American Psychological Association.

Brennan J, Hollanders H (2004). Trouble in the village? Counselling and clinical psychology in the NHS. *Psychotherapy and Politics International 2*(2): 123–134.

Debord G (1994). *Society of the Spectacle (*Nicholson-Smith D, trans). New York, NY: Zone Books.

Grant B (1990). Principled and instrumental nondirectiveness in person-centered and client-centered-therapy. *Person-Centered Review 5*(1): 77–88. Reprinted in Cain DJ (ed) (2002). *Classics in the Person-Centered Approach.* Ross-on-Wye: PCCS Books (pp371–376).

Illich I (1976). *Medical Nemesis: the expropriation of health.* New York, NY: Pantheon Books.

Miller SD, Bargmann S, Chow D, Seidel J, Maeschalck C (2016). Feedback-informed treatment (FIT): improving the outcome of psychotherapy one person at a time. In: O'Donohue W, Maragakis A (eds). *Quality Improvement in Behavioral Health.* Cham: Springer International Publishing (pp247–262).

Newnes C (1999). Histories of psychiatry. In: Newnes C, Holmes G, Dunn C (eds). *This is Madness.* Ross-on-Wye: PCCS Books (pp7–27).

Orne MT (1962). On the social psychology of the psychological experiment: with particular reference to demand characteristics and their implications. *American Psychologist 17*(11): 776–783.

Proctor G (2018). *The Dynamics of Power in Counselling and Psychotherapy: ethics, politics and practice* (2nd ed). Monmouth: PCCS Books.

Rogers CR (1976). Interview with Professor Anthony Clare. *All in the Mind.* BBC Radio. Cited in: Sanders P, Hill A (2014). *Counselling for Depression.* London: Sage Publications.

Rose N (1985). *The Psychological Complex: psychology, politics and society in England, 1869–1939.* London: Routledge & Kegan Paul.

Sanders P (2005). Principled and strategic opposition to the medicalisation of distress and all of its apparatus. In: Joseph S, Worsley R (eds). *Person-Centred Psychopathology: a positive psychology of mental health.* Ross-on-Wye: PCCS Books (pp 21–42).

Sanders P, Tudor K (2001). This is therapy. In: Newnes, C, Holmes G, Dunn C (eds). *This Is Madness Too.* Ross-on-Wye: PCCS Books (pp147–160).

Ware P (1983). Personality adaptations. *Transactional Analysis Journal 13*(1): 11–19.

World Health Organization (2018). *International Classification of Diseases and Related Health Problems* (11th revision). Geneva: WHO.

3 | Psychiatry: a dangerous raft in a sea of despair

Sally Fox

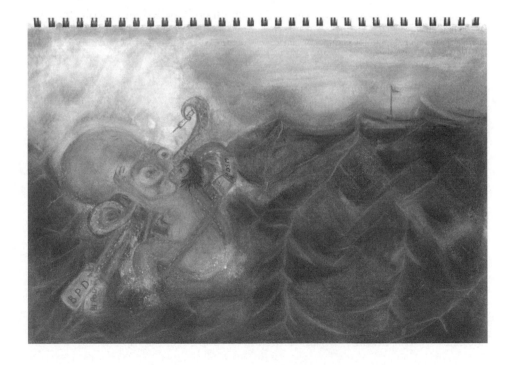

This chapter was first written as an assignment for the Mad People's History and Identity course run by CAPS Advocacy and Queen Margaret University in Edinburgh, which I took in 2016. The requirement was to describe in 1,000 words an image that illustrated an aspect of the course that resonated with us.

I was struck by a painting by the artist Helen Flockhart called *The Encounter* and used it in my assignment as a metaphor to explore how helpful psychiatry was in dealing with distress. Here, I use my own image and experience of psychiatry.

The image shows a human desperately clinging to an octopus – a creature that is familiar with the sea (its environment), but not an obvious companion to guide her to the safety of the shore. There is a marker in the distance, but the subjects are stuck, treading water in a co-dependent clasp.

The sea represents mental distress, the octopus psychiatry and the marker is the flag raised when primary care can no longer manage the distress and provides a referral. In the image, the octopus is the only refuge in the sea, much like psychiatry in the business of mental health, and its grip can be likened to the eight tentacles of a beast that both rescues and entraps.

Tentacle 1 – referral

I, and I suspect many others, had mixed feelings about being referred to psychiatry. I found it validating to know that my distress was being taken seriously, but in conflict with this was the fear that I'd be sectioned, labelled and medicated like my mother, who had died young and in a 'mania'.

Tentacle 2 – diagnosis

We are presented with a *fait accompli* model of disease arising from chemical imbalance and faulty genes. Within 20 minutes of being seen by a psychiatrist, I was told my 'symptoms' were evidence of the 'bipolar illness' I had inherited from my mother. There was no room for negotiation or support to relate and make sense of my distress in terms of my life experience, even though that was the help I was seeking. It felt like I was being objectified and silenced.

Tentacle 3 – medication

Consistent with a biomedical paradigm, medication was the obvious and first choice of treatment for me, and for most service users. Contrary to popular belief, psychiatric drugs don't target specific symptoms; they deaden all affect – joy as well as sadness. So-called 'side effects' often intensify and compound the problem, leading to further health complications, diagnoses and drugs. Despite being troubled by 'a rash, shakes, gastric irritation, liver dysfunction and rapid weight increase' (as detailed in my notes, and I am talking about gaining three stone over three months), I was deemed to have 'excellent compliance'!

Tentacle 4 – psychological therapies

Inflated with a cocktail of prescribed toxins, I could float in denial for a while, supported by monthly blood tests and the 'mood stabilising' clinic, which seemed to back my diagnosis's tenuous link with science.

My referral to psychology was deemed inappropriate because of the time commitment I would require and the view – again, as expressed in my notes – that I would 'disadvantage others on the waiting list'. I was offered, as a poor substitute, psycho-education classes on depression, anxiety, self-esteem and assertiveness. A mere 10 weeks of art therapy on the NHS barely touched the source of my pain. What it did do was reveal my difficulty in building trusting relationships, which the system was woefully inadequate to rectify.

Tentacle 5 – attachment and trauma
For me, and I believe for most people who present to psychiatry, unresolved trauma and attachment issues from childhood were at the root of my distress and were distorting my ability to deal with it effectively. In terms of how psychiatry responds, this might as well be the invisible tentacle. The neglect and poor treatment we receive (in the form of short-term interventions, frequent changes of staff, constantly being seen through a sick lens) reactivate and exacerbate the original trauma and rejection. The longer you are held in the system, the more persistent its effects.

Tentacle 6 – prognosis
On reflection, being given a diagnosis is a minefield of medication, side effects, over-dependence and inter-relational traps, as well as the damage that comes from being labelled as the problem. For those who remain in the clutches of psychiatry for long, the prognosis is poor.

Tentacle 7 – discharge
Being released from the tentacles of the beast presents a precarious challenge: will we sink, or will we swim? Personally, I found discharge a daunting prospect, but it made me more resourceful and resolute in finding the help I had originally asked for. For others, it can be the first of many exits and entries back into services.

Tentacle 8 – label
Arguably the most tenacious tentacle is the label you are left with. No matter where you are on your personal journey of recovery or self-discovery, others will continue to see you through the filter of your diagnosis and it becomes their default when treating or relating to you, even if the label no longer applies. Unfortunately, you will not find the removal of a label recorded in your notes, which is where the frequently used comparison of a broken leg diverges from mental 'illness'. A broken mind seems to imply a broken soul that permeates the person's judgement and core values.

Conclusion

Drawing on the literature I've read and my own personal case notes, I cannot find any conclusive evidence to justify and sustain our current biomedical understanding and treatment of mental distress. So, to return to my analogy of clinging to a vessel in a sea of despair, psychiatry, while arguably doing its best to prop us up, is simply the wrong raft. Those very tentacles reaching out to save us increase the probability of drowning.

Further, I would suggest that stigma is a product of psychiatry, because it insists on labelling, objectifying and isolating people and their reactions to distressing life events, whether current or historical. Stigma is the shadow of the asylum, the birthplace of diagnosis, with its roots in 'moral treatment'.

Psychiatry has failed to evidence its organic theories and yields ever-more 'mental disorders', published in successive versions of its so-called bible, the *Diagnostic and Statistical Manual of Mental Disorders* (*DSM*) (American Psychiatric Association, 2013). It is time to ditch the octopoid raft.

Perhaps society would understand and be more empathic if 'madness' were presented as the result of life trauma. It wouldn't be as frightening as the unpredictability of 'mental illness' framed as a biological epidemic affecting more and more of the population.

Life can be brutal and it can be beautiful. An understanding of resilience and attachment, along with a trauma-informed approach that acknowledges a person's own story, could create the foundations for a relation*ship* that is fit for purpose and can help us navigate seas of calm and despair.

Reference

American Psychiatric Association (2013). *Diagnostic and Statistical Manual of Mental Disorders* (5th ed). Washington: APA.

4 | The revolution will not be pathologised

Dolly Sen

I had a Sunday ritual that many British teenagers in the 1980s shared with me: I would record songs from the radio, hoping that I wouldn't get the DJ's voice intruding on my tape. It was an escape from the pain that was all around. My mind had nowhere to rest, to be safe, nowhere to find peace. Aged 14, I had already endured over a decade of serious physical, emotional and sexual abuse and neglect, along with nearly losing two siblings to serious illness. My only sanctuary was school. I loved it. I was academically gifted and enjoyed the work. Aged 12, I was voted by my class the person most likely to be successful. But by age 13 I had to deal with a new agony: bullying at school. My As became Bs and Cs; I was losing concentration and motivation. My dad tried to improve my school grades by attempting to strangle me.

What could my mind and endlessly breaking heart do but seek reprieve in small ways like music? But this particular Sunday, the music was interrupted by a demonic voice laughing and saying things like 'What do you want?' At first I thought it was radio interference, so I unplugged the radio, but I could still hear the voice. I then thought, 'Oh my god, the devil is speaking to me.' It was soul-destroying and terrifying, but I didn't have parents I was able to confide in. Besides, the voice told me this was between me and him, otherwise he would kill my siblings in the most horrific ways. Some minutes later, the voice disappeared. But the next day it returned and has not left me since, more than 30 years later. As the week wore on, more voices came into that lonely, broken room, and I was seeing shadows following me. The last straw was seeing a demonic face over my shoulder when I looked in the mirror while brushing my teeth. I took an overdose to escape this hell. I survived. I felt sick and my stomach hurt so much, but I was living and breathing still. The voice said, 'You can't escape me now.'

I withdrew at home. I refused to go to school because I thought people there were going to kill me. Social services got involved because of this and referred me to see a child psychiatrist at my local hospital in south London. I was so nervous meeting her but was also desperate to speak to someone about what was happening. I wanted someone to stop me drowning. When I stepped into the consulting room, I was not thrown a lifeline or life preserver but a concrete block. The first thing she said to me, without even making eye contact, was, 'So what's wrong with you?' It was a heartbreaking thing to say to me. What was WRONG with ME?

The psychiatrist had a checklist of questions and I felt myself shrink smaller and smaller with every question. I seemed to be an annoyance to her, a waste of her time. She asked me really personal questions, such as ones about abuse, with such coldness in her voice, it made me want to kill myself there and then. So, she became another person to add to the list of people who didn't care, who couldn't protect me, and another reason not to trust. Just in case I couldn't get that, she ended the session by telling me to 'pull up my socks and stop being silly'. It was hard to even entertain that notion when I thought demons were chasing me. My meeting with her didn't convince me that hell didn't exist. Funnily enough, I didn't want to engage with her, or the tens of psychiatric workers that followed who shamed my mind by calling it disordered, aberrant, abnormal.

I have had a few different diagnoses over the years. It started off as 'depression', then 'psychotic depression', then 'schizophrenia'. After that, it was 'bipolar', and now it's back to 'psychotic depression.' Not one of those labels did me any good. The medication has been the same, the not being listened to has been the same, the shame and powerlessness have been the same. Having so many different labels also puts paid to the idea that diagnosis has scientific validity. After all, I have had no biological test in the last 30 years of my 'care'. These diagnoses come from value-based subjectivity of what is acceptable in society. Psychiatry is not an objective science; nor does it value the subjectivity of its patients. By looking objectively at the most subjective of experiences, which is what psychosis is, things will get lost or missed; stories that need to be voiced get untold, and it just becomes a mirror that holds the face of a vilifying, unkind, systematically abusive so-called medicine. Physician, do no harm – unless you are a psychiatrist; then it is part of your remit. And these days we have psychologists placed in job centres, forcing people to be more positive or they will lose their benefits, and ignoring the socio-political impacts on people's mental health. This once kinder discipline is following down the slippery slope of its older counterpart.

So what can I thank diagnosis for? Well, it helped with getting benefits when I was at my most unwell, but if I had been given real help as a 14-year-old

I probably would not have needed them. If I put my diagnosis on my business card, I would be guaranteed to lose out on a job 99 times out of 100. Oh, let's not forget the time I was sexually assaulted when I was an inpatient and, when I told a nurse, was told it was all in my head, because that's what my diagnosis means.

As psychiatry didn't help, I had to find other ways to cope. Luckily, I discovered creativity, such as writing and art, which helped me express difficult feelings. I wrote poems about loneliness that made me feel less lonely. I realised I was drawing myself a map. If services and systems provide you with a map on how to be lost and stay lost, you need to find the map elsewhere. Creativity has done that for me. It is also a great way to explain what being a diagnosed, pathologised human being feels like. Here are a couple of poems that do just that.

Dignity cannot be taken four times a day

Being labelled, pathologised and medicated,

I cannot claim my mind for myself

I cannot claim my life for myself

So how can I even have dignity?

Medicine does not heal

But seals the scream

Is that dignity?

Dignity is never in the side effects.

Weight gain – my arse is getting bigger than my dreams.

Too tired to reach for the day, let alone the sun.

Try having sex without coming – dignity?

Love with a lot of going – dignity?

A journey of a thousand miles starts with a single step, but try it with a largactyl shuffle.

Constipation does not feel like dignity

How can I sing the song of dignity, drooling?

I would walk away with my head held high, but am too tired, too alone, too despised.

But let's put aside the pills for a moment.

Is dignity in the waiting room?

Is it in the set of eyes that sees you as a sickness?

How much does dignity cost exactly? It's not in our budget this year. It's not in the economic case.

Dignity is not in the control and restraint, face down, begging to breathe.

It was not in the staggered silence of my 'community care'.

It is not in the 'burden of care' phrase.

I am still waiting for my appointment with dignity.

Dignity means not begging for my identity, my dreams, it means not
    begging to be heard, to be cared for.

Dignity means honouring the person, but not being hated will do.

Dignity cannot be taken four times a day.

And shouldn't be bitter pills to swallow…

Maybe this little poem called 'Shame on the mental health service' will help some
professionals see the invisible monologues they have with their 'patients'.

Shame on the mental health service

Tell us your shame.

Tell me your most shameful secrets.

You are not going to tell me?

Then you must be sick.

You need treatment.

You need my expertise.

My expertise means I can have no shame.

I can hide it.

But you must always tell me yours when you see me.

Must I restrain you to protect me from myself?

Here, have more shame to drown you.

You must engage.

You must engage in your shaming.

I don't know why you are not getting any better.

Psychiatry and society say I should be ashamed for hurting because of trauma,
ashamed that I am mad. What is diagnosis except a less-than label, a lack of
compassion, fairness, a lack of love? There's something deeply wrong with
psychiatry. It takes deeply hurt people and aims to numb them out of their
humanity or hurt them more by using disgusting language to make their
souls feel small and their hurt feel larger, or uses physical force, alienation or
indifference.

Maybe I can drive home the message by taking well-known quotes about
love and giving them a psychiatric twist. Here goes!

All you need is love. But a little chocolate now and then doesn't hurt.
(Charles M Schulz)
All you need is love. But a little control and restraint to force you to take drugs doesn't hurt. (Psychiatry)

Love is that condition in which the happiness of another person is essential to your own. (Robert Heinlein)
Love is that condition in which the happiness of another person must be pathological. (Psychiatry)

There is no remedy for love but to love more. (Henry David Thoreau)
There is no remedy for love so let's increase your medication until you can feel no love. *(Psychiatry)*

There is only one happiness in this life, to love and be loved.
(George Sand)
There is only one happiness in this life, to love and be loved… unless you are mad. Then you don't deserve it. (Psychiatry)

Love doesn't make the world go round. Love is what makes the ride worthwhile. (Franklin P Jones)
Love doesn't make the world go round, because the earth is flat! (Psychiatry)

Love notes from psychiatry are prescriptions of pain and shame and desolation. They do not taste sweet.

Looking back, I have some anger over those encounters, and I wonder how my life might have been different if I had met warm, kind, supportive professionals who didn't break me by calling me broken. Maybe my life would have played out the same, but I know I would have experienced a little less pain. But what if I had met someone who didn't think there was anything wrong with me, who could see I'd been hurt and reduced that hurt, not added to it? Instead, I lost my youth and my 20s to extreme mental hell, and psychiatry added to that pain whenever I met it. Psychiatrists medicated me but that left me lost behind a fog; my trauma became an eerie but distant presence but it didn't go away. Madness might mean my mind is at war with itself but psychiatry has made me a refugee from my own soul. Most mental health difficulties are not about broken brains but broken hearts. And I had to carry this heart and its broken pieces around with me until I was 30.

I finally found my way into some kind of light in my 30s. If you, like me, have been residing in psychotic hinterlands for a good few decades, you realise, when you rejoin society, you are decades behind your peers. Your first love, job, career, home, relationships are new things in your 30s and 40s.

People talk of lost youth like a misplaced item. Mine was never there in the first place. Another thing to thank psychiatry for.

When you stumble with mistakes in middle age that most people dispensed with in their teens, it's humiliating and demeaning. It skins you alive when you have no skin to begin with. Your vulnerability feels like a coat of petrol in a world of fire. It adds shame to more shame.

So, I see arts as an opportunity to develop ways to reclaim my identity from a mercenary, judgemental world that has abused it. The sanitised world insults my dreams and humiliates my soul. Asking me to be normal is asking too little of me; it asks too little of all of us.

The British artist Nigel Henderson said that art is the battleground for the human spirit. And tablets do not mend a broken heart. Creativity knows the heart needs love, that it needs a new story and should be respected and be exceptional.

You need to free your mind twice; before you tackle mental pain, you have to free yourself from psychiatry. Label yourself creative thinker rather than broken mind. Too many of us are given the message that our inner realities, our very selves, are pathological and must be hidden. Too many of us feel like lesser beings. How can we be lesser if we can, through creativity, make our lives as bold and colourful and beautiful as we like? That is what creativity is: the power to change.

Let's not beat around the bush: psychiatry has defined your mind as ugly, but why do you see your mind as ugly when I see the beauty of it? Why are other people owning your definition? Who says you are you? Who has written your script? If you don't like your script you are living, write a new one. If you don't like the people around you, recast the characters. I realised this for myself. I realised I was giving my narrative on a plate to those who couldn't even write a pot noodle ad. Also, I think 'psychosis' is a story/experience that can't be told in its purest form. Creativity can help that with its gentle re-writing. Psychiatry does not understand gentle re-writing. It understands the heavy, brand stamp that wants to crush you into wellness.

I have used art to rewrite my story and have taken the liberty of re-writing the *Diagnostic and Statistical Manual of Mental Disorders* through the medium of sheep. I love sheep, I love humour and I love art, so I have combined the three to show that paradigms can be shifted in very few words. It only needs the will of the people who work within the system to put it into practice.

The *Diagnostic Sheep Manual* frames an experience to put the sheep in a hurtful and alienated position. The shepherd is looking for the sheep to be herd but not heard, to prepare it for existential slaughter.

On the next page is an example of how it does that.

But actually, the flock alienated the black sheep for being different; the badge of 'black sheep' comes from others, it is rarely self-defining. Don't ewe see that it is unscrupulous to alienate someone for difference and then insist they change

THE BLACK SHEEP
or social disengagement histrionic disorder

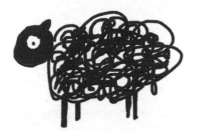

Symptoms

- Flaunts difference
- Refuses to dye fleece to fit into the flock
- Attention-seeking and self-centred

Treatment of social disengagement histrionic disorder

BLEACH FLEECE WHITE

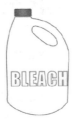

- Side effects: can cause sores, fleece loss, low sheep-esteem
- But hey, you fit in now

colour to relieve the rest of the flock's discomfort? Wouldn't it be better to:

- accept that it is OK to be different and we shouldn't fear it?
- not isolate others?
- not label difference?
- know a black fleece is just as warm as a white fleece?

Here is another example.

THE LOST SHEEP
or obsessive disorientation disorder

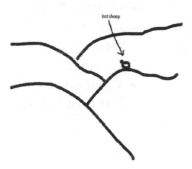

Symptoms

- Disorganised thought
- Inflexible about orientation
- Pervasive pattern of lostness
- Attention-seeking (wants to be found)

Treatment of obsessive disorientation disorder

- Chaining lost sheep
- Electronically tagging lost sheep

Side effects

- Obesity from lack of movement
- Apathy (if you can't go very far, why go at all?
- Arrest for absconding can cause death or trauma

Instead, why not give the lost sheep a map? Or map-reading skills? Or signposts that actually point to useful places? Why not provide a packed lunch? Or understand that not all who wander are lost?

The mental health system I would like to see

First, it must throw away compliance and coercion as gods. The alternatives must aim not only to depathologise but to change the world that causes so much distress. It must fight against the psychocompulsion, the benefits and services cuts. It needs to be political. After all, if compassion isn't a political act in this world we reside in, what is?

Second, I would like there to be no need for this disclaimer:

> You do not have the right to say anything without it being used against you. Anything you say can and will be used against you. You have the right not to use these services. If you do not use these services, you will lose your benefits and then your home. Do you understand the rights I have just read to you? With these rights in mind, do you wish to engage in our therapeutic relationship?

I'd like us to be able to talk openly and honestly with each other without fear of turning those words into wounds, whether the wound is a label, unkindness or coercion.

Through absorbing neoliberal values of the system, through training, through working the machinery of pathology, how can we expect our mental health workers to be kind? It is taken from them, because kindness can mean someone going, 'Whoa, why are you forcing meds on a person? Why don't you address their insecure housing, their abused lives and their lost place in society?' Kindness means not decontextualising people's lives to fit into boxes. It means their biography belongs to them and isn't yours to rip into and assault with pathology. It means not rejecting their stories. It means gently helping them re-write their stories into what those stories should have been.

Those who don't share a downgraded status need to ask themselves, how can I help the person maintain dignity? How can I help them be neither passive nor aggressive in a world that looks down on them? How can I help them explore what really hurts them, in a safe and meaningful way? Or how can I change institutional discrimination, given that this institution pays my salary? Difficult questions, yes. But, as we keep getting told by therapists, change is painful.

I would like the mental health worker to be more humane. I, as a patient, am expected to share what shames; I am expected to be vulnerable. The worker is protected from that. I am not protected from the demeaning, humiliated position that puts me in. Either the space is there for both of us to share equally, or psychiatry has to find ways not to shame us and make us feel more vulnerable when we step into the consulting room.

I would love it if there were no need for psychiatrists to have power over the broken person. A hurt person does not need someone who has more power over them. They need compassion. And I don't mean compassion as a personal approach to the person. I mean compassion in doing their part to change the system they are working in. If enough people who work in the system refuse to collude, it has to change. Please don't tell me how hard that will be, because I know it from experience. I have had a few years training in occupational therapy, which means I have been on placements in clinical settings. I had to challenge colleagues about bad practice or make a complaint about someone's behaviour (for example, I reported a psychiatric nurse who said, 'The only thing you can do with people with personality disorder is drop a chair on their head') so often that none of my co-workers, who were there to teach me how to work as a clinician, would speak to me. I was alienated, rejected. It only took one person to be on my side for there to be power in that action and for me not to feel shame and upset about doing the right thing.

I would love any therapy to be individualised to suit the person. It's possible, because I had a psychologist who did that for me. She gently and warmly individualised the therapy so it was meaningful to me. I love all animals, but sheep especially, so she turned my schema therapy for 'psychosis' into 'find my inner sheep' therapy. She turned my dissociation into a lost sheep and my sense of being evil into a black sheep, so I could relate to it better and so I could learn to be a kinder shepherd to my broken heart. She was more of co-conspirator than a medical professional, and I am forever grateful for her input to my life. But I also know she couldn't be as open within the system as she was with me, and that's half the problem. And her role meant she couldn't use it to challenge social and political inequalities – that's another part of the problem.

The mental health system is such a tangled mess, that much is obvious. Other than three people among the hundreds of workers I have met, the mental health system has beaten me internally into a pulp. I have become weakened by it. If I ever take my own life, they have helped me on my way there, and it all starts with turning my pain into a 'disorder' that individualises the distress within me, and not a response to what has happened to me. It all begins with 'What is wrong with you?' and not 'What happened to you?' It begins with: 'You have a broken brain, not a broken heart, so now it doesn't matter if we break that heart further, and we will.' I say, 'Drop the disorder, drop the diagnosis and elevate and respect that broken heart.'

Until things do change, I will be an activist. I will fight for the broken hearts. Activism is challenging stereotypes, countering bullshit, creating personal and community armour, rejecting our place in the world, gnawing at injustice and engaging in our own liberation, whether psychically or physically, or even poetically.

The revolution will not be pathologised
No forced stillness and wiped dreams
No being held down
For being different
No sedation for the screams
We are screaming for a reason
Our hurt will change the world
Because the world won't change our hurt
The side-effect of life
Is the need for it to be ours
The revolution will not be medicated
You cannot anaesthetise hell
You cannot desensitise the broken heart
It needs to be brought off its knees
To stand tall
Over everything that has broken it.
If you can't make it stand,
You have to fall.
The revolution will not be pathologised.

5 | Problems in living: an existential perspective

Emmy van Deurzen

Life is rarely easy and for many people it becomes distinctly problematic at some point during their lifetime. It is hardly surprising that four out of 10 people struggle with mental health problems. It has been habitual over the past 100 years to treat such problems as medical issues and to deal with people's emotional and existential difficulties by prescribing medication, but there is more and more evidence that this is not the best response. It is high time that we dared to deal with problems in a more direct manner and use our understanding of human existence to tackle them. This is something I learnt the hard way through my 45 years of working in mental health and I hope that my experience may be of some benefit to those who are currently struggling with this issue.

Personal discoveries

I was raised in the 1950s and 1960s, in the Netherlands, by parents who were theosophists and homeopaths, at that time a rarity, and I was taught to be cautious about medical interventions very early on. When a serious road traffic accident at the age of 10 landed me in a coma in hospital, where I had to remain for an extended time, this caused me many troubles and difficulties. I felt overwhelmed and scared of the technology surrounding me, especially when I was subjected to hours of old-fashioned, hard-core radiography of my head, not knowing what was going on but hearing people speak about hairline fractures of the skull and wondering if I would be OK.

I was at the same time grateful for the care and safety that was created around me, in a darkened, quiet room. But I was constantly terrified of what they were going to do to me. I had become very fearful and anxious after the accident and nobody provided me with any kind of guidance. My parents were only allowed to visit me rarely and briefly. Having had a near-death experience and being left flat on my back in an isolated room for long periods of time, I had much to think about. I wasn't allowed to read or play in any way and I became adept at reflecting on myself and the other people around me. The experience changed me profoundly and I began to desperately yearn for love and freedom and to make something meaningful of my so nearly destroyed but now miraculously restituted life.

I wanted to help other people and change the world for the better in some way. I was aware of all the suffering in the ward across from my glass windows. I became impatient to get through my education. I no longer wanted to be a child, at the mercy of other people's rules and regulations. I wanted to strike out in the world and find my own mission and project. Eight years later, I left the Netherlands as soon as I had finished my final exams and went to Montpellier, in the south of France, to study philosophy. I wanted to understand all about human existence.

My French boyfriend, who was soon to become my first husband, was a medical student who began specialising in psychiatry months after we met. I went to many of his psychiatry lectures and started volunteering alongside him as he worked first as an extern, then as an intern, at the city's psychiatric hospital, Font d'Aurelle. This was the main psychiatric teaching hospital in the Languedoc region, and it was an educational experience to work there on voluntary placement between 1971 and 1973. My initial background for my work here was as a philosopher with some training in psychoanalysis, including a short period of personal therapy.

Safeguarding and disarming

My first confrontation with psychiatry came as a shock. I worked half-days in the children's ward and was initially appalled to see how kids and adolescents with 'autism', learning difficulties and all manner of other psychiatric diagnoses were kept in this locked, chaotic, noisy country house, which was set within vast and impressive grounds, among the other wards of the hospital. It was a universe all of its own. There was a separate locked area for non-verbal and non-ambulant children with genetic disorders. They were mostly under 10 years of age, as they rarely survived their first decade. They were hugely disabled, often physically as well as mentally. They cried in distress and many seemed in pain, despite high levels of sedation. They were penned in cots, sometimes chained to the rails. Their parents rarely visited them, or any of the other children on the ward for that matter, but medical experts came from all over the world to observe, examine and study their rare conditions. It felt wrong and sinister, like a living museum of human deformity.

The one good thing was that experienced specialist nurses looked after these children and seemed very dedicated and caring. It brought back my own memories of lying in my isolated bed in the hospital at the age of 10, when kind nurses looked after me. My heart went out to these children, knowing there would be no cure for them and no new departure. They were trapped inside dying bodies. Sometimes it made me weep and I would be berated for this. I was told I was too soft hearted. This idea was anathema to me. It seemed to me we needed more, not less humanity in the midst of this disturbing and upsetting situation. I was no less perturbed by the way in which the ambulant kids were penned in with each other in the central courtyard of the ward all day. Many of them wore scant or no clothing, as they tended to rip fabric to shreds in a matter of minutes or hours. About half of them wore helmets to protect their skulls from frequent head banging and they could be seen standing by walls or in door jambs exercising that small privilege of sensory experience afforded by the repeated clanging.

My contribution to the ward was mainly to take the most able of the ambulant children for walks around the extensive grounds of the hospital or play with them in the front garden of the children's ward. I tended to avoid the dismal courtyard. I had a natural gentleness and empathy that made it easy for me to befriend them and I particularly enjoyed taking them to see the chickens and pigs at the other end of the hospital grounds. Such outings would take several hours, with all the stops on the way and picking up of sticks and stroking of hens and collecting of eggs for an omelette. The children all loved going on these outings and, although they were non-verbal, they showed their pleasure in multiple ways, by cooing and smiling, wild rocking, excited whooping and flapping of hands. They often showed affection too, a keenness to hold hands or grab my shirt or stroke my hair. This was in the days when it was quite acceptable to hug the kids right back.

There were some children who were lacking in emotional expression and who avoided all such contact. They were often the most wide-eyed and best-looking ones, mute and too well-behaved for their own good. Shocking events had traumatised them and they were lost in a nightmarish world of their own. Some heard voices or might suddenly become fearful and stubbornly unco-operative if thwarted. Stories of their childhood trauma were whispered around the ward in hushed tones by the nursing staff. I had very little trouble with them, because I was able to let them be and they sensed my forbearance and knew I was no threat. Others were challenging and noisy and quick to violence. I had to learn to manage them, which was a learning curve I initially found hard but rapidly took in my stride, nevertheless. One of them, Luc, a lad of 14, was severely autistic and non-verbal, but confidently vocal and often aggressive with the younger ones. His face showed the early down of puberty and, although he was a head shorter than me, he was built a great deal more robustly and was quite a lot stronger. It was a good thing that there had to be at least two staff members on every outing of eight children.

I watched how different nurses and carers managed the children differently. Each had found their own way of dealing with the difficulties they posed and I learnt a lot from each of them. I was keen to get better at managing Luc in particular, as he had a way of turning on the other kids maliciously and viciously, setting off a chain reaction of protest and panic. He was also well known for attacking staff whenever possible. In the beginning he used to grab hold of my arms, when given half a chance, and twist the skin on my forearm sharply, drawing blood or bruising me. The nurses would laugh at my beginner's gullibility. I learnt to steer clear of his kicking, scratching and punching. My Judo skills came in handy on several occasions, when I was able to show him my strength and capacity to control him. He learnt to behave himself sensibly with me, because he relished the outings more than anyone. He was able to cluck like a hen and snort like a pig and he revelled in the exercise and the company.

I was well aware that Luc was in the habit of throwing nasty temper tantrums, which were bewildering in their violence, and I wanted to make sure I would know how to deal with such a situation if it happened on a walk. So, I discussed the best way of handling Luc with a small group of nurses. One of them claimed to have the most effective method of controlling Luc and he went on to proudly demonstrate it. This nurse, whom I shall call Georges, was in his early 30s and had a reputation for being fairly macho. He rode a large motorbike and wore leathers, and always had a cigarette between his lips, even when he was riding. This was not too surprising, as most people in psychiatric hospitals smoked in those days. Cigarettes were often used as a form of payment and exchange between staff and patients. Male patients were even given a tobacco allocation.

Georges traded in cigarettes like a gang master and this in itself gave him an aura of power over the young male patients. But now he showed us a different way of using his smoking habit, as he ordered Luc to go get his packet of cigarettes from the table. When Luc predictably refused to oblige and started protesting vociferously, Georges ran after him, caught him with a certain amount of panache and proceeded to burn Luc's lower arm, cruelly and insistently, with his lit cigarette, telling him he should obey him next time. Luc ran away in terror, howling. Some of the other nurses were as shocked as I was. Others were quite casual about it. Using burning cigarettes as cattle prods may have been new to me but it was clearly an old trick as far as some of them were concerned. I had noticed that Luc's arms were covered in scars but had been told that this was the result of his self-harm. Indeed, I had previously seen Luc hold his own arm on a stove, while loudly laughing about it, until 10 minutes after. I was horrified and immediately understood that when Luc was pinching the skin on my own forearms, he was giving me burns, passing on the very suffering he was so afraid of.

Georges argued that some amount of violence was the only way of keeping Luc under full control. He was not ashamed or contrite when some of his colleagues disapproved and told him to stop doing this if he didn't want to be reported. He maintained it was a clever device and an acceptable thing to do when faced with Luc's viciousness. Georges accepted that it caused distress to Luc, who would often go on to throw a tantrum in consequence. But, far from this convincing him that it was the wrong thing to do, he just smiled and said this was part of the technique, as when Luc had a violent tantrum Georges would phone the psychiatrist on call to get an emergency prescription for an injection of stronger sedatives. Then he would have an easier time with the children for the rest of the day. He said it was the only way to keep Luc under control when he was alone on the ward on night duty.

The debate about Georges' conduct did the rounds of the team for many weeks and there was by no means unanimity about it. Many took the view that, with a patient like Luc, who was like a wild, wilful animal, strong measures were sometimes required. There were general discussions with the team about morals and professional etiquette and, as a result of the entire episode, Luc's daily dose of sedatives was raised considerably, which certainly made for greater calm in the service almost immediately. Soon after this episode, Georges asked for a transfer to a different ward. Some lessons had clearly been learnt and private talks had happened between him and the head of the team.

I continued thinking about this episode for a long time. It taught me to be more modest in my judgements about medical treatment. I appreciated that, if I had had the daily task of dressing Luc or taking him to the toilet when he had messed his pants, I might have been less inclined to hold the same moral high ground as I did in my position as young volunteer who didn't carry any real responsibility. I became aware of the clash between the morals we hold in theory and the ones we apply in practice. I also became aware that the nurses had learnt to see their young patients more as animals than as human beings and that this allowed them to be more casual and detached than I was. The decision to put Luc under heavy sedation made good sense to all of them. I was the only person who was pleading for a gentler approach. I continued to hold this perspective and felt sorry for him as he lost his usual vibrancy and was no longer able to come for walks. He now spent most of his time sleeping or dozing or sitting on the floor of the dayroom or in the courtyard, rubbing his genitals. All this left me feeling much more aware of the huge challenges in psychiatry. I accepted that many of the staff saw their role as one of safeguarding rather than educating, let alone curing their patients.

People like Luc didn't stand a chance. They were dehumanised by the severity of their condition. They were caught in the vicious circle of their own diagnosis and the way they were treated made them worse and worse. They were merely kept from harm, not treated. The older nurses told me many stories about the old days before psychoactive medication and I began to see the great advantages of the new drugs in terms of easing the tension for carers. Patients who were incapable of language and could not manage socially acceptable behaviour did not have a say. The objective of the system was to stop them harming themselves and others and keep them under control. I began to read more and more Foucault to make intellectual sense of what was happening (Foucault, 1963, 1965, 1973). I realised that people like Luc were given up on from the start. I often thought about our friendly walks and his enthusiasm for the pigs and chickens. I regretted I had not been able to do more for him and I knew that, despite the difficulty, this might have been a possibility had I been more experienced and in a position of authority. I knew for sure that we could have done better for Luc than we did, and I knew I wanted to work somewhere where I could learn about this.

The medicalisation of impotence

Soon the rotation moved on and now I became involved in an entirely different ward: the acute unit for young women, in the same hospital. These patients were largely young or middle-aged, depressed, anxious and suicidal women. Some had eating disorders. None of them had learning difficulties or 'autism'. There were long discussions about whether each of them was 'neurotic' or 'psychotic', 'hysterical' or 'schizophrenic'. Again, this was a shock to me, for these seemed to me like ordinary women, just like me or the women who worked as nurses or care assistants. I felt an immediate affinity with them, especially the younger ones. To me, at this time, psychiatric care became very suspect: it became a question of feminism and liberation against the mostly male medical establishment. I was quickly cautioned not to fall into over-identification. But identification was the only way in which I was able to really understand and empathise with these patients. I have continued to use that principle throughout my later years as a therapist. If I can't find a way to identify with a person, I simply cannot get a handle on their predicament. The challenge always is to identify with the person first and then to find the strength to face their challenges with them. Identification without the inner strength and clarity to overcome problems is worthless sentimentality. But treatment without identification and empathy lacks in understanding and sensitivity. It was from Karl Jaspers' work that I first learnt to allow myself to fully participate in my clients' experiences (Jaspers, 1963).

The women I met at this ward taught me this lesson. I felt outraged when they became upset at the treatment meted out to them and their reaction was interpreted as more evidence of their 'mental illness'. But I knew that mere resonance with their plight and a capacity to feel their pain were not going to be any good to them either. They were often quite passive, and I knew that the challenge was to enable them to regain the power that they had given away. I wanted to advocate for them, but soon realised that this was far from helpful to them. It just confirmed them in their role as patients. They were generally given benzodiazepines or antipsychotics, depending on whether they were diagnosed as 'neurotic' or 'psychotic'. The dosage of their medication was increased regularly as long as they were complaining, crying, isolating themselves or not eating. When they stopped self-harming and ceased protesting, started eating and fitted in with the ward routine, doing embroidery or knitting in the dayroom with the other women, they were left alone and usually discharged soon. If they remained suicidal after several weeks of treatment, they were prescribed ECT without hesitation.

I found all this troubling in the extreme and in a much more personal way than the problems I had encountered in the children's ward. These young women were often intelligent and very capable. To me, they were ordinary people who had had bad experiences. I wanted to speak with them and help them resolve their problems. I could see that they all started out feeling terribly agitated and became increasingly submissive and confused by their medication. I observed that this was seen as the treatment, that they were expected to calm down and stop bothering people. I could tell that they were worried about having been assigned the role of 'mental patient'. They often started dismissing themselves for being 'mentally ill' or crazy. They would initially claim not to be able to speak with me because they were not intelligent, saying to me that they were useless or ill or incapable of solving any problems. I was reminded of the way in which the children in the other ward were treated as animals and saw now how these women were also dehumanised and objectified. They were treated as second-class citizens in such a way that they ended up believing they were incapable and incompetent. Most of them had fallen between a rock and a hard place: they didn't want to be a mental patient, but nor did they know how to cope, actively and effectively, with their situation on their own. They frequently said things to me like: 'What can I do? What can I say? Others will decide what is best for me.' I wanted them to take charge of their lives, but still had to learn how to teach them to do so.

Despite my strong feelings, my role was mostly that of a friendly companion, encouraging the women in their embroidery or persuading them to come out of their rooms to join in with the others. I wasn't allowed to provide any therapy yet, but occasionally I was able to persuade one of the women to come for a walk around the grounds. The outdoors and the physical exercise would shake them up immediately and they would start speaking in a different voice. They became friendly and quickly trusting and we could talk about what lay behind their suffering. These conversations did not come under the mantle of psychotherapy, which was mainly given by the psychoanalysts. My conversations with these women were ordinary, friendly dialogues conducted with great ease as part of a casual outing. I was only 21 years old, but I had been through some pretty tough times in my life, which I have written about elsewhere (van Deurzen, 2015). The younger women trusted me without question, especially the ones who were fasting. I was rather skinny, and it was obvious that I had neither the authority nor the desire to try to trick them into eating.

I remember Sylvie in particular. At 17, she had tried to hang herself in her father's barn and had been hospitalised in a coma. Since then, after returning home, she had stopped eating and now, at 18, had been sectioned as she was considered to have a malignant obsession with self-destruction and dying. She had been force-fed, like a goose, she said. She was pretty fierce and very angry. Nobody had really allowed her to express these feelings. Nobody was interested in her side of the story. Her dad had told the police she was mad, and something had to be done about it. Her psychiatrist had told her that she needed to obey her parents' rules; she was grown up now and had to contribute to the family farm. She had always helped out in the past with smaller jobs but had left school at 16 when she was expected to take charge of various jobs on the farm she didn't want to do.

She told me with disgust about the fattening of pigs for slaughter. She also described in great detail to me how pigs would scream when they were slaughtered. I already knew a thing or two about that. She had no intention of changing her mind and she was prepared to die rather than being part of her father's bloody industry. But, to her parents, she was insane for refusing to eat the very food that was their livelihood. Sylvie had no idea what else she could do. Despite her strong views, she had no positive plans for the future. She had not worked any of it out in her own mind. She had just learnt to say 'no' to them when she felt disgusted. She had stood her ground, she felt, but then they had won the battle by declaring her mad. And she had begun to think they must be right about that.

She realised as she was talking about it with me that perhaps if she was going to be saying 'no' to so many things in her life, she also needed to decide which things she was going to say 'yes' to. Sylvie was puzzled about this idea of saying 'yes' at first and said she had never really thought about it. Her experience was black and white. She thought she would either have to accept her father's rules and continue living at home or say 'no' to the rules and end up being a mental patient. It was her against the world. Not eating was a way of registering her disagreement, but it had turned into self-sacrifice, a martyrdom that was killing her. All her energy had gone into not being fattened up like the pigs and not collaborating in the work on the farm that would lead to the death of her animals. As she saw it, it was either the animals dying, or her. I pointed out that right now it was both the animals and her that were dying.

She started telling me all about her life now. The pigs and geese had always been her best friends and she had to do something to show her loyalty to them. She had not found a better way to oppose her father's trade than to do so by self-destructive action. She felt bad about living off his money. She knew that her refusing to eat ham and sausages had really got to him. It was the best she could do; at least he had been forced to take notice of her. I asked her to think of ways in which she might find a better solution to her predicament that did not involve her killing or depriving herself. She then admitted she didn't really want to die and that she often secretly ate the stale bread meant for the pigs. She was puzzled by what her Lacanian psychoanalyst-psychiatrist had told her. His interpretation of her situation was that she was 'denying the law of the father' and that this demonstrated her inability to accept the rules of society. She did not really understand what he meant by that. All she wanted to do was to stop her father killing the animals she was attached to.

She saw herself as a heroine rather than as a mental patient initially, but she did realise that her father's 'law' had now won as he had been able to get her locked up. She feared she would end up a mad woman. She knew she could not win the battle between them, but she promised me she would think of ways in which she could say 'yes' to something, so that she could find a positive goal. I mentioned I was a vegetarian and that perhaps she could commit to that regime without feeling she was giving in too much. Sylvie left the hospital just a few days later, having started eating again. She had declared herself a vegetarian. People had accepted that compromise. This was my first small therapeutic success, but it was not followed up. Sylvie simply left the hospital and I never heard from her again.

Finding an existential phenomenological solution

It was deeply frustrating to me to have so little authority in these situations and I found it upsetting to watch these women fighting so many losing battles that I could not help them with. My now husband and I often discussed these things and he thought me very naïve for arguing that there was nothing wrong with his patients. He was training to be a psychiatrist and he was learning to measure his power and responsibility as a medical practitioner. It was hard for him to think we might be witnessing social, cultural and political issues rather than medical ones. It was then that we both started reading Laing (1959, 1961, 1967) and Szasz (1961), making us both more radical. But it was in coming upon Binswanger's case studies that our discussions about the meaning of these patients' predicaments became more in- depth and specific. Binswanger had tried to understand young women like Ellen West and Susanna Urban (Binswanger, 1963; May, Angel & Ellenberger, 1958) without attributing their predicament to mental illness. Jaspers' work on psychopathology added a new dimension as well (Jaspers, 1963). We now decided to find a place where we could work together in a way that would allow for such an approach to psychiatry.

Meanwhile, I had become a serious student of the work of the existentialists, reading most of Sartre's books and finding them very relevant (Sartre, 1985, 2001/02, 2003). Camus' (2005) descriptions of the human condition were also vivid and helpful, especially in understanding alienation. I found Simone de Beauvoir's work particularly helpful, as she spoke in the female voice, so often suppressed. I immediately resonated with her autobiographic novels, as well as with her theoretical work in *The Second Sex* and *The Coming of Age* (de Beauvoir 1970, 1973). It gave me the courage of my own convictions and enabled me to seek a different way to engage with the women I worked with. Now I began thinking of therapy as a form of liberation and empowerment and began calling myself an existential therapist, seeing myself as researching the vagaries of the human condition.

My husband and I studied the social experiments that had been happening in France at Saint Alban and Laborde, in Italy at Gorizia and in Belgium in Geel.

I avidly read Jan Foudraine's book *Not Made of Wood* (Foudraine, 1974) when it came out in Dutch in 1971. We attended a year-long seminar on community psychiatry and learnt all about the English experiments at the Northfields and Cassel hospitals and the experiments at Chestnut Lodge in the US. We visited most of these places ourselves over the years. Saint Alban was by far the most intriguing, as it was located relatively near Montpellier. I was aware of the work of psychiatrists Georges Daumezon and François Tosquelles, who had revolutionised the old asylum there, and we had the privilege of meeting a now retired Daumezon and his wife in their house in the Cevennes. He strongly recommended we should take the risk of living and working in Saint Alban. We took up the challenge and applied for jobs.

The hospital was well known among the French psychiatric community in the early 70s, as it had been the first mental hospital where the walls were taken down at the end of the Second World War. It had become the most famous place for experimentation with the therapeutic community model through the 1950s and 1960s. It had lost its status of cutting-edge innovation, as this had shifted to La Borde Hospital. Nevertheless, Saint Alban was a revelation to me. The hospital was based in the heart of the Massif Central, a mountainous area in central France, that had serious snow for several months of the year. It was built around a medieval castle, which had been turned into a workhouse, then into an asylum. A decade previously, film-maker Mario Ruspoli had shot his documentary *Regards sur la Folie* (*Views on Madness*) there, based on the work of Artaud and Foucault (1963, 1965, 1973). It was amazing to live and work there.

Now, in the early 1970s, the hospital was well established in its alternative modality, with freedom for most patients (easy to do, they told me, because nobody would be foolish enough to run away from a hospital that was so isolated in the countryside). Every person who was able worked and everyone had therapy. Additionally, we found a community spirit that was unmatched by anything I have ever come across elsewhere. The hospital staff were, at that time, closely engaged with the patients and often spent a portion of their free time socialising with them as well. In fact, the village of Saint Alban had 2,000 inhabitants and 700 of them were patients and most of the others were nurses or nuns (whose community was central to the hospital), or people running local shops and services. Hospital life was based around ergo-therapy and socio-therapy. This meant that everyone in the hospital did something to earn their keep. This might be helping on the ward or in the kitchens; working in the commercial printing press, which produced books and posters; working in the wood carving and furniture workshop, which produced handmade tables, sculptures, spoons and bowls and many other objects to an extremely high standard; working in the pottery, which produced mugs and coffee and tea pots, or in the hospital hairdressers, beauty shop or dress makers, on the hospital radio or in its film and photography studios, or in the canteen, workshop, pharmacy or bar. Others were employed in the shop or the gardens or garages. Many were helping local farmers and in the autumn some would travel to wine-growing areas to help with the grape harvest in local vineyards. It all was pretty overwhelming and impressive. The social club was located at the centre of it all, on the castle square. It offered continuous, day-and-night entertainment and therapeutic engagement and was considered to be the heart of the hospital and its communal mission.

I was proud to be offered a job at the club, which had only four full-time employees. I was given a psychologist post and was expected to replace the wife of the last consultant, who had just left. My husband, newly qualified, replaced him, and although we were so much younger, we were expected to fill the immense vacuum they had left. They had both been experienced group psychotherapists. My three colleagues at the club told me they would show me the ropes and they did, indeed, teach me all they knew over the nearly two years I worked with them.

I immensely enjoyed my work in Saint Alban (see van Deurzen 2010, 2012, 2015; van Deurzen & Adams, 2016), and relished the little extras, like taking patients out for Easter-egg hunts, or going skiing, or having wonderful village fêtes, for which the patients prepared all sorts of stalls and gave performances. I even learnt to referee the Petanque competitions on these occasions. I sometimes worked with patients at the radio station and became very involved in psychodrama sessions. A special stage had been built for this purpose and many of the staff had been trained in the method. I mixed my psychodrama with philosophy and learnt on the job, drawing the line at making Lacanian interpretations, which was the favoured sport of many of the others.

I had amazing conversations with people from all sorts of backgrounds. Some had done dreadful things, like killing a family member or a politician, but all of them wanted redemption and understanding. I was never frightened and always felt safe and protected in this community. I learnt to listen to people's fears as much as to their hopes for a decent life and future. I learnt to accept their madness and find their humanity. Most of these people taught me invaluable lessons – far more, I am sure, than I ever taught them. In fact, it was by listening to their stories and their feelings and by helping them to find clarity and distill their wisdom that I learnt my profession of existential therapy.

References

Binswanger L (1963). *Being-in-the-World* (Needleman J, trans). New York, NY: Basic Books.

Camus A (2005). *The Myth of Sisyphus* (O'Brien J, trans). London: Penguin Modern Classics (first published 1942).

De Beauvoir S (1973). *The Second Sex* (Parshley HM, trans). New York, NY: Vintage Books (first published 1949).

De Beauvoir S (1970). *The Coming of Age.* (O'Brian P, trans). New York, NY: Putnam.

Foucault M (1973). *I, Pierre Riviere, Having Slaughtered my Mother, my Sister and my Brother* (Jellinek F, trans). New York, NY: Pantheon.

Foucault M (1965). *Madness and Civilization: a history of insanity in the age of reason.* New York, NY: Random House.

Foucault M (1963). *The Birth of the Clinic* (Sheridan A, trans). London: Tavistock Press.

Foudraine J (1974). *Not Made of Wood: a psychiatrist discovers his own profession* (Hoskins HH, trans). London: Quartet Books.

Jaspers KA (1963). *General Psychopathology.* Chicago, Il: University of Chicago Press.

Laing RD (1967). *The Politics of Experience.* Harmondsworth: Penguin.

Laing RD (1961). *Self and Others.* Harmondsworth: Penguin.

Laing RD (1959). *The Divided Self.* Harmondsworth: Penguin.

May R, Angel E, Ellenberger HF (1958). *Existence.* New York, NY: Basic Books.

Sartre J-P (2003). *Being and Nothingness: an essay in phenomenological ontology* (Barnes HE, trans). London: Routledge (first published 1943).

Sartre J-P (2001/02). *The Roads to Freedom* (*The Age of Reason, The Reprieve, Iron in the Soul*) (Sutton E, Hopkins G, trans). London: Penguin Modern Classics (first published 1945/49).

Sartre J-P (1985). *Existentialism and Human Emotions.* New York, NY: Citadel Press (first published 1957).

Szasz TS (1961). *The Myth of Mental Illness.* New York, NY: Harper Collins.

van Deurzen E (2015). *Paradox and Passion in Psychotherapy* (2nd ed). Chichester: Wiley.

van Deurzen E (2012). *Existential Counselling and Psychotherapy in Practice* (3rd ed). London: Sage.

van Deurzen E (2010). *Everyday Mysteries: existential dimensions of psychotherapy* (2nd ed). London: Routledge.

van Deurzen E, Adams M (2016). *Skills in Existential Counselling and Psychotherapy* (2nd ed). London: Sage.

6 | Deceived: how Big Pharma persuades us to keep taking its medicines[1]

James Davies

Over the last 10 years, criticism of psychiatric diagnosis has grown in both volume and credibility. Taking as an example the controversy surrounding the 2013 publication of the *Diagnostic and Statistical Manual of Mental Disorders* (*DSM-5*) (American Psychiatric Association (APA), 2013), in that year alone more than 100 critical editorials, op-eds and articles were published in the broadsheet media, alongside an array of articles in prestigious academic journals such as *Nature* (Ledford, 2012); the *British Journal of Psychiatry* (Bracken et al, 2012) and *The Lancet* (2012). These variously charged *DSM-5* with over-medicalising human suffering by lowering diagnostic thresholds and expanding the number of 'mental disorders' with which people can be diagnosed. These and other criticisms that have been levelled against previous *DSM* editions (Kirk & Kutchins, 1992; Caplan, 1995; Kutchins & Kirk, 1997; Davies, 2016; Greenberg, 2013; Kirk, Gomory & Cohen, 2015) gained unprecedented professional support in late 2012, when more than 50 mental health organisations internationally (including the British Psychological Society, the American Psychoanalytic Association, the Danish Psychological Society and the American Counseling Association) signed an online petition calling for a halt to the publication of *DSM-5*.[2]

During that same period, many critical books also drew public attention to the severe problems of psychiatric diagnosis more broadly (for example, Paula

---

1. This chapter was previously published in slightly altered form in the following book: Vos J, Roberts R, Davies J (2019). *Mental Health in Crisis*. London: Swift Sage. It is published here with kind agreement of the publishers.

2. The petition can be viewed at www.ipetitions.com/petition/dsm5

Caplan's denunciation of 'Psychiatric diagnosis as a last bastion of unregulated, rampant harm to the populace' (2013); *The Book of Woe* (Greenberg, 2013); *Cracked* (Davies, 2013); *A New Prescription for Psychiatry* (Kinderman, 2014), and *A Straight Talking Introduction to Diagnosis* (Johnstone, 2014). In sum, these works, in various ways, highlighted the unscientific manner in which diagnostic manuals and tools are contrived and deployed, the poor reliability and validity of psychiatric diagnosis, the endemic conflicts of interests between *DSM* committees and the pharmaceutical industry, and the stigma (both public and self-stigma) that psychiatric labels invariably induce.

As I write this, in 2019, the critical momentum has not abated, with books, articles and public debate continuing to flood public and professional discourse and mental health professionals and users/survivors, often in coalition, coming together in national and international organisations and movements to challenge the diagnostic frame (for example, the Global Summit on Diagnostic Alternatives;[3] the Drop the Disorder! campaign,[4] the Power Threat Meaning Framework[5] and the Hearing Voices Network[6]). These initiatives are actively developing, evaluating, advocating and disseminating alternatives to current diagnostic thinking and practice. In short, the burgeoning international criticism of the making and assigning of psychiatric labels is no longer confined to a small subset of intellectuals and survivors previously dismissed as 'antipsychiatrists'; it now constitutes a mainstream and authoritative social movement, such is the conviction in large sections of the mental health, media, survivor and service-user communities that the medical model of mental distress is failing those in need.

The purpose of this chapter, then, will be to revisit some of these critical arguments and to articulate some new ones. In particular, I shall focus on what Robert Whitaker has referred to as the 'economies of influence' (Whitaker, 2017) – those conflicts of interests (financial and professional) that have aided diagnostic expansion in recent decades and, thus, the over-medicalisation and medicating of our behavioural and mental states. In short, if we are to move beyond the current biomedical paradigm of emotional distress to embrace more effective non-medical alternatives, then identifying the failings of our current approach is a necessary first step.

The construction of diagnostic manuals

Diagnostic manuals such as the *DSM* and the World Health Organization's

---

3. See http://dxsummit.org (accessed 25 June 2019).

4. www.adisorder4everyone.com (accessed 25 June 2019).

5. www.bps.org.uk/news-and-policy/introducing-power-threat-meaning-framework (accessed 25 June 2019).

6. www.hearing-voices.org (accessed 25 June 2019).

equivalent, the *International Classification of Diseases* (*ICD*) (WHO, 2018), have expanded the number of mental disorders over consecutive editions. In the last 35 years, the *DSM* has more than doubled the number of mental disorders believed to exist, from 106 in the 1960s to approximately 370 today.[7] In addition, the diagnostic thresholds people must meet to receive a diagnosis have also been progressively lowered, resulting in more types of suffering being captured by diagnostic criteria today than at any other time in the past. Taken together, these processes have led to what is called 'diagnostic inflation', or 'over-medicalisation' – namely, the unjustified reclassification of many natural and normal (albeit painful) human responses to the problems of living as 'mental disorders' requiring medical intervention.

Such diagnostic inflation did not emerge from any advances in biological research (there are still no known biomarkers for nearly all 'mental disorders'), but rather from the consensus-based and culturally situated judgements of small and deliberately selective groups of *DSM* and *ICD* committee members. Research has exposed the highly arbitrary and culture-bound processes by which diagnostic systems were contrived and expanded by such committees (Carlat, 2010; Davies, 2013, 2016; Kirk & Kutchins, 1992; Caplan, 1995; Kutchins & Kirk, 1997; Greenberg, 2013; Kirk, Gomory & Cohen, 2015). In the absence of any guiding neurobiological research, and in the face of mostly contradictory and incomplete clinical data, small diagnostic committees throughout the history of psychiatry have essentially relied on reaching consensus among themselves about how disorders should be defined, where to set diagnostic thresholds, and whether to add or remove diagnoses. Archival and oral histories of how such consensus was formed, at least during the construction of the *DSM*, have paid careful attention to the processes leading to committee consensus. This research has shown that committee voting was a central mechanism by which key *DSM* conclusions were decided about how to define 'disorders', whether or not to include them, and where to set the thresholds for receiving them (Davies, 2017).

While it goes without saying that voting is not a scientific activity, some may argue that the more recent editions of *ICD* and *DSM* were based on more scientifically robust processes. While this argument has been regularly advanced, there remains no evidence to substantiate it. One reason for this is that the processes governing the construction of later manuals – such as *DSM-5* – still remain opaque in areas, despite some excellent work by Greenberg (2013). (For example, members of the *DSM-5* task force were asked to sign confidentiality agreements by the publishers, the APA, prohibiting them from discussing DSM's construction after the fact.) Furthermore, the APA has embargoed all materials pertaining to the construction of *DSM-5* for 15 years post-publication, making any

---

7. The figure of 370 is arrived at by counting the main in-text categories and their sub-divisions, as well as all appendix inclusions. These are counted because they are all categories with which people can be diagnosed.

objective assessment of its construction impossible to undertake.) Furthermore, even if the argument could be made that latter processes were more robust, it is important to note that the construction of *DSM* is a cumulative process (each consecutive edition building upon the last). Therefore, most inclusions ratified by vote in 1980s still live on in *DSM-5* today.

The psychiatric drug crisis and epidemic

While it is, therefore, right to discount *DSM* and *ICD* as credible works of science (they are works of *psychiatric culture*, not of science), we can take the critique further still by showing how these cultural artefacts have inflicted significant harm. They harm not only by stigmatising the human propensity to suffer (suffering is no longer a natural and understandable human protest, but a 'biomedical disorder' of the self) but also, due to the over-medicalisation caused by diagnostic inflation, by driving vast increases in psychiatric prescribing since the 1990s (Béhague, 2009). Such has been the success of the medicalisation/medicating regime that in many industrialised nations (including the UK and US) more than 20% of the adult population has been given a psychiatric drug prescription in the last 12 months (Smith, 2012; Duncan & Davis, 2018).

To understand the specifics of this figure, and focusing on antidepressants alone, more than 7.3 million people were prescribed antidepressants in England in 2016–17) (Hansard, 2018). This constitutes 16% of the entire English adult population – with the number of individual annual prescriptions now topping 65 million (NHS Digital, 2017). But it's not only prescribing rates that are increasing; so too is the average length of time that people spend on the drugs, which has doubled since the mid-2000s in the UK (NHS Digital, 2017). Today, around half of all people taking antidepressants in England (3.5 million people – or eight per cent of the adult population) are taking antidepressants long-term – that is, for longer than two years (Johnson et al, 2012).

As to why antidepressants are being taken for longer periods, this can be partly explained in the light of new evidence revealing that our current guidelines on antidepressant withdrawal (NICE, 2009 and APA, 2010) significantly underestimate the commonality, severity and duration of the adverse effects people experience when trying to stop taking the drugs. This underestimation can lead to withdrawal reactions being misdiagnosed as, for example, relapse (the return of the original symptoms), and drugs being reinstated as a consequence (Davies & Read, 2018; Breggin, 2007). This state of affairs is both upsetting and bemusing, given it suggests many people are becoming trapped on drugs that are, for most of them, no more effective than placebos, and only show very minor (ie. clinically insignificant) improvements over placebo for the most severely distressed (Cipriani et al, 2018). In short, for most people the differences between placebo and antidepressant are clinically insignificant. However, unlike placebos, antidepressants elicit side effects for between 40–70% of people taking them, as well as withdrawal effects for around 50% – effects that, by being misdiagnosed or not tolerated, are fuelling longer durations of use of the drugs.

Rising long-term antidepressant use is of serious concern. Alongside the obvious economic costs, the human costs are more serious, as long-term use is associated with increased severe side effects, the impairment of autonomy and resilience (increasing a person's dependence on medical help), increased weight gain, worsening outcomes for some people, poorer long-term outcomes for 'major depressive disorder', greater relapse rates, increased mortality and an increased risk of developing neurodegenerative disease, such as dementia (Davies & Read, 2018).

When we turn to antipsychotics, the situation is similar. Their long-term use is associated both with increased risks of serious adverse cardiovascular, metabolic, and neurological side effects (Salvo et al, 2016) and with decreased social functioning and worsening symptomatology (Harrow & Jobe, 2007; Harrow, Jobe & Faull, 2012). For example, the first randomised controlled trial (RCT) to compare continued antipsychotic use with tapered withdrawal after 18 months showed that, after seven years, the withdrawal group had much better functioning and twice the rate of recovery than the long-term-use group (Wunderink et al, 2013).

Research showing the harms of long-term use is crucial when realising that, wherever we are seeing longer and more widespread use of such drugs, mental health disability claims are increasing too. Over the last 20 years, rates of mental health disability in the UK have doubled, and similar disability increases are seen across the developed world (in Australia, Iceland, the US, New Zealand and Sweden, for example). In other words, wherever psychiatric drug use is rising, disability rates are rising too (Whitaker, 2016).

The fact that we can observe this correlation across different countries (all with different health systems, levels of inequality, welfare provision etc) obliges us to consider the extent to which the adverse effects of the drugs themselves – particularly antidepressants – are fuelling the rising global burden of mental health disability. Given the importance of these considerations, as well as the harmful effects psychiatric drugs can clearly elicit, it is vital to critically assess how drug consumption is being fuelled by medicalisation on the one hand and its aggressive industrial promotion on the other.

Industry influence on medicalisation

How then does the relationship between medicalisation and rising psychiatric drug consumption actually operate? What mechanisms of influence does the pharmacological industry exert to expand drug consumption via medicalisation? Putting it in the least varnished terms: how do pharmaceutical companies influence processes of medicalisation to aid the wider consumption of their products?

In order to address this question head on, it will be useful to first distinguish between two forms of industry influence – *direct* and *indirect*. In the first case, *direct* influence denotes the undertaking of activities explicitly designed to increase psychiatric prescribing, such as direct marketing and advertising initiatives. As this type of influence is clear in both form and intent, and as its effects have been extensively covered elsewhere (Angell, 2011; Smith, 2005; Lacasse & Leo, 2005), I shall restrict myself here to focusing on its more clandestine alternative: *indirect* industry influence. This latter process broadly denotes a form of financial influence that is harder to spot – one that invariably operates by proxy and/or purposeful default, such as the financial sponsoring of people, institutions and apparatuses deemed sympathetic and/or potentially advantageous to the expansion of psychopharmaceutical markets.

An obvious example of indirect influence is the financial sponsorship by the pharmaceutical industry of 'key opinion leaders' in the mental health and psychiatric fields. When researchers at the University of Massachusetts inspected the financial interests of the 'experts' who sat on the various committees of *DSM-IV*, they exposed the extent to which this kind of influence permeates our diagnostic systems. Of the 170 people constructing *DSM-IV*, 56% (95) had one or more financial associations with the pharmaceutical industry; of those on the committees that decided the 'disorders' for which drugs are the first-line treatment, 88% had financial ties to drug companies (Cosgrove et al, 2006; see also Caplan, 2008).

This form of indirect influence is so immensely powerful because it is accepted as typical and routine within the psychiatric profession – a normalisation that seems to have inoculated many against perceiving the true depth of its biasing effects. An example of such normalisation was powerfully illustrated to me at a debate in the UK Houses of Parliament in June 2013, when I raised the issue of industry payments with the chair of the task force that put together *DSM-IV*, Allan Frances. He acknowledged that, while the *DSM* committee essentially comprised 'good guys' who wanted to do a good job, maybe it was remiss that *DSM-IV* did not have a conflict-of-interest policy at the time it was developed; in the 1990s, he explained, such financial ties were not deemed relevant enough to warrant declaration.

While *DSM-IV* had no conflict-of-interest policy, the later edition, *DSM-5* (APA, 2013), certainly did. This was partly due to other areas of medicine, during the mid-2000s, exposing the biasing effects such conflicts generate and advocating for total transparency. Following this trend in medicine more widely, transparency was introduced to *DSM-5*. The result was that, of the 29 people on the task force charged with writing the manual, 21 were revealed as having previously received honoraria, consultancy fees or funding from pharmaceutical companies, including the chair, David Kupfer, and the vice chair, Darrel Regier (Davies, 2013).

While those possessing financial ties to the pharmaceutical industry often dismiss or downplay the biasing effects, research reveals a very different conclusion – that they prejudice recipients (both institutions and individuals) towards favouring psychopharmaceuticals in their clinical, educational and research activities (Orlowski & Wateska, 1992; Lexchin et al, 2003; Adair & Holmgren, 2005; Lo & Field, 2009; Spurling et al, 2010). Given that *DSM* has medicalised swathes of painful normality and driven up drug prescriptions as a consequence, it is concerning that those responsible for such over-medicalisation were financially linked to the very companies set to benefit from this vast expansion of drug consumption that over-medicalisation has engineered (Whitaker & Cosgrove, 2015; Davies, 2017).

My second example of indirect influence relates more specifically to diagnostic practices in the UK's National Health Service (NHS), and in particular to two of the most influential mental health diagnostic tools administered in UK – the patient questionnaires PHQ-9 and GAD-7. From the mid-2000s, these documents began to be used throughout primary care to enable GPs to assess whether a person has 'depression' (PHQ-9) or 'anxiety' (GAD-7) and, if so, how severely.

A major criticism of PHQ-9 and GAD-7 is that they set a very low bar for what constitutes having a form of 'depression' or 'anxiety' for which a drug should be prescribed. For instance, if you indicate on PHQ-9 that in the 'last two weeks' you have 'nearly every day' experienced poor appetite, troubled sleep and low concentration and energy, you qualify for the diagnosis of 'moderate depression', which, according to NHS guidelines, is sufficient grounds for prescribing an antidepressant. This low threshold becomes more concerning when we discover that PHQ-9 and GAD-7 were developed, their NHS distribution paid for and their copyright owned by Pfizer Pharmaceuticals – a company that makes two of the most often prescribed anti-anxiety and antidepressant drugs in the UK, Efexor (venlafaxine) and Zoloft (sertraline).

Allowing a pharmaceutical company to set the clinical thresholds for the prescribing of their own drugs is an exemplary example of how indirect industry influence works.

My final example of indirect influence draws on a personal anecdote. During a research trip to New York City in November 2013, a colleague drew my attention to the fact that the number one best-selling book in the US at that time (according to Amazon's top 10 list) was *DSM-5*, and that it had been within the top 10 for six months since its publication in May that year. To get a sense of scale, this ranked it alongside the Harry Potter books and *Fifty Shades of Grey*, also recently published. Also, DSM-5 was hardly cheap, with the paperback version costing $88 a copy. So why were so many people buying it?

I raised this question the following day in a meeting with a professor of psychology at New York University. She worked in primary care in the New York State area and had discovered the reason why DSM sales were so high was because the pharmaceutical industry had been buying copies in bulk and distributing it free to clinicians up and down the state (a practice that, she ventured, was occurring nationwide). For her, why the industry would do this was obvious: 'As almost any kind of suffering is caught by the *DSM*, disseminating *DSM* is just good business: it drives up diagnosis rates and, with this, prescriptions.'

While the above illustration still remains to be definitively verified,[8] it is consistent with other indirect methods whereby the pharmaceutical industry has historically promoted psychiatric drugs, especially with respect to their targeting of academic and clinical professionals in order to drive up prescription rates. Since the 1990s, for example, the pharmaceutical industry has been a major financial sponsor of UK and US academic psychiatry, significantly influencing psychiatric research, training and practice (Carlat, 2010; Whitaker & Cosgrove, 2015; Gøtzsche, 2013). Many heads of psychiatry departments receive both departmental income and personal income from drug companies (Campbell et al, 2007); nearly all clinical trials of psychiatric drugs (antidepressants, neuroleptics, tranquillisers) are financed by the industry (Angell, 2011); most academic drug researchers receive research funding, consultancy fees, speakers fees or other honoraria from the industry, and leading psychiatric organisations, such as the American Psychiatric Association (the publisher of *DSM*), receive most of their operational costs from the industry (with this support, the APA's annual revenues rose from $10.5 million in 1980 to $50.2 million by 2000 (Whitaker, 2017; Davies, 2017)).

That pharmaceutical companies have actively used their extensive financial power to shape practice and ideology within the mental health field will surprise no one. But the extent to which these companies have promoted over-medicalisation (ie. they have concertedly targeted how we think about human distress in order to normalise psychiatric prescribing) is still not fully appreciated. Anthropologists, in particular, have demonstrated in great detail how pharmaceutical companies have purposively translated local, non-medical languages of distress into Western, medicalised, *DSM*-based nomenclature in order to actively create new markets for their products (Kirmayer & Minas, 2000; Skultans, 2003; Ecks, 2005). The anthropologist Stefan Ecks called this process 'metaphysical globalisation' (2005), where the dissemination of *DSM* and *ICD* classifications in new locales becomes an essential step in expanding psycho-pharmaceuticals into new markets.

Another anthropologist, Vieda Skultans (2003), has analysed 'metaphysical globalisation' in operation. Taking Latvia as an example, she showed that, following the translation of *ICD* into Latvian, pharmaceutical companies undertook and funded large campaigns to 'educate' Latvian psychiatrists and family doctors about the new diagnostic category of 'depression'. This led to the gradual reconceptualisation of a local understanding of distress – *nervi* – into the Western category of 'clinical depression'. The concomitant shift in

---

8. Six months after this exchange, I was undertaking research in the *DSM* archives at the American Psychiatric Association in Arlington, Virginia. While there, I was interested in verifying this statement. However, even though the archivist did confirm that most sales of DSM were indeed bulk purchases, I was also told that the APA was unable to gather 'customer-end' information.

practice (from investigating the possible social and political meanings of *nervi* to treating 'depression' pharmacologically) led to *nervi* being depoliticised and reconfigured as a medical problem, which opened up a brand-new market for antidepressant drugs.

Similar mechanisms were analysed by Junko Kitanaka (2013) and Ethan Watters (2011) in Japan, during GlaxoSmithKline's (GSK) marketing of its SSRI antidepressant Seroxat in the early 2000s. At that time the Japanese description of mood that came closest to depression, *utsybyo*, described a chronic illness that was as severe as 'schizophrenia' and for which people needed to be hospitalised. Therefore, large swathes of the less severely distressed, who would be prescribed SSRIs in Europe and the US, fell outside the pool of consumers that companies could psycho-pharmaceutically target. As a result, GSK undertook a directed campaign to convince these untreated people to think of their varied forms of moderate distress not only as 'depression' but also as something that was treatable with Seroxat. TV adverts were funded to market the condition to the public and some 1,350 Seroxat-promoting medical representatives visited selected doctors on average twice a week, priming them to prescribe Seroxat to the coming influx of 'depressed' patients (Schulz, 2004). 'Depression' websites and web communities were also established by GSK, while being made to look like grassroots movements. As a result, the category of 'depression' won wide cultural salience and Seroxat sales rose to $200 million in the two years following the campaign (Davies, 2013).

While I offer only two examples above, similar processes have been observed by anthropologists in China, Argentina, Chile, India and elsewhere, prompting Kirmayer and Minas (2000) to propose that the global spread of psychiatric disease classifications and diagnostic processes can help account for the vast global increases in antidepressant use (Ecks, 2005). Pharmaceutical companies would probably respond to these criticisms by arguing that these promotional activities – both at home and abroad – are justified on the grounds that they advance healthcare to people who would otherwise be denied effective treatment; that by educating populations into the virtues of the medical management of emotional/social/psychological distress, their promotional activities both at home and abroad perform a vital public and human service.

Of course, where psycho-technologies genuinely help the distressed, these arguments have some currency. However, research has shown that the safety and efficacy of psychiatric drugs in particular have been vastly exaggerated by both industry and those professionals whom industry funds, and that growing consumption of such drugs has been driven less by their clinical success than by good marketing concealing bad science (Smith, 2005; Lacasse & Leo, 2005), the manipulation and burying of negative clinical trials data (Kondro & Sibbald, 2004; Turner et al, 2008; Spielmans & Parry, 2010; Angell, 2011), lax medicines regulation (Healy, 2006), poor provision for non-drug alternatives, and strong financial allegiances between industry and psychiatry (Campbell et al, 2007; Cosgrove et al, 2006; Timimi, 2008). In short, the argument that pharmaceutical promotion has placed sufferers' needs before the interests of the industry's shareholders is difficult to substantiate.

Conclusion

In this short chapter I have briefly outlined certain dynamics linking pharmaceutical industry influence, the over-medicalisation of suffering and the over-prescribing of psycho-pharmaceuticals. If I were to trace a causal chain of events, the first factor – industry influence – enables all that follows, which, from the standpoint of industry, is precisely the point: such influence is a costly investment from which a return is expected (a return that can only result from increasing diagnoses and prescriptions). While industry influence drives medicalisation and over-prescribing, it would be wrong to ignore the fact that the pharmaceutical industry itself is only able to wield such influence because the flimsy legislative checks and balances on its activities allow it to do so. In short, wider sociological analyses as to what enables such *carte blanche* influence are essential in understanding why nearly 20% of our adult population is psychiatrically medicated at any given time.

To understand the drivers of this prescribing epidemic, we must move beyond assessing the interests and practices of psychiatry and the pharmaceutical industry (as important as they are) to also inspect the systemic political/economic arrangements that allow such interests to thrive, despite worsening clinical outcomes from these drugs and growing evidence of the harm they can do (Davies, 2017). In short, the current biomedical crisis is not just to do with over-medicalisation and over-prescribing, and the evident harms of each, but also with the factors that permit these processes to operate unchecked in the health sector worldwide (Kirk, Gomory & Cohen, 2015).

References

Adair RF, Holmgren L R (2005). Do drug samples influence resident prescribing behavior? A randomized trial. *American Journal of Medicine 118*(8): 881–884.

American Psychiatric Association (2013). *Diagnostic and Statistical Manual of Mental Disorders* (5th ed) (DSM-5). Washington: APA.

American Psychiatric Association (2010). *Practice Guideline for the Treatment of Patients with Major Depressive Disorder* (3rd ed). Washington, DC: APA. https://psychiatryonline.org/pb/assets/raw/sitewide/practice_guidelines/guidelines/mdd.pdf (accessed 30 July 2019).

Angell M (2011). The illusions of psychiatry. *The New York Review of Books 58*(12): 82–84.

Béhague DP (2009). Psychiatry and politics in Pelotas, Brazil: the equivocal quality of conduct disorder and related diagnoses. *Medical Anthropology Quarterly 23*(4): 455–482.

Bracken P, Thomas P, Timimi S et al (2012). Psychiatry beyond the current paradigm. *British Journal of Psychiatry 201*(6): 430–434.

Breggin P (2007). *Your Drug May Be Your Problem: how and why to stop taking psychiatric medications* (revised ed). Cambridge, MA: Perseus Books.

Campbell EG, Weissman JS, Ehringhaus S et al (2007). Institutional academic-industry relationships. *The Journal of the American Medical Association 298*(15): 1779–1780.

Caplan PJ (2013). Psychiatric diagnosis as a last bastion of unregulated, rampant harm to the populace. In: Dellwing M, Harbusch M (eds). *Krankheitskonstruktionen und Krankheitstreiberei: die renaissance der soziologischen psychiatriekritik*. Wiesbaden: Springer (pp351–388).

Caplan PJ (2008). Pathologizing your period. *MS Magazine* (summer): 63–64.

Caplan PJ (1995). *They Say You're Crazy: how the world's most powerful psychiatrists decide who's normal*. Reading, MA: Addison Wesley.

Carlat D (2010). *Unhinged: the trouble with psychiatry*. London: Free Press.

Cipriani A, Furukawa TA, Salanti G et al (2018). Comparative efficacy and acceptability of 21 antidepressant drugs for the acute treatment of adults with major depressive disorder: a systematic review and network meta-analysis. *The Lancet 391*(10128): 1357–1366.

Cosgrove L, Krimsky S, Vijayaraghavan M, Schneider L (2006). Financial ties between *DSM-IV* panel members and the pharmaceutical industry. *Psychotherapy and Psychosomatics 75*(3): 154–160.

Davies J (ed) (2017). *The Sedated Society: the causes and harms of our psychiatric drug epidemic*. London: Palgrave Macmillan.

Davies J (2016). How voting and consensus created the *Diagnostic and Statistical Manual of Mental Disorders* (DSM-III). *Anthropology and Medicine 24*(1): 32–46.

Davies J (2013). *Cracked: why psychiatry is doing more harm than good*. London: Icon Books.

Davies J, Read J (2018). A systematic review into the incidence, severity and duration of antidepressant withdrawal effects: are guidelines evidence-based? [Online.] *Addictive Behaviors*; 4 September. https://doi.org/10.1016/j.addbeh.2018.08.027 (accessed 26 June 2019).

Duncan P, Davis N (2018). Four million people in England are long-term users of antidepressants. [Online.] *The Guardian*; 10 August. www.theguardian.com/society/2018/aug/10/four-million-people-in-england-are-long-term-users-of-antidepressants (accessed 25 July 2019).

Ecks S (2005). Pharmaceutical citizenship: antidepressant marketing and the promise of demarginalization of India. *Anthropology and Medicine 12*(3): 239–254.

Gøtzsche P (2013). *Deadly Medicines and Organised Crime: how Big Pharma has corrupted healthcare*. London: Radcliffe Publishing.

Greenberg G (2013). *The Book of Woe: the DSM and the unmaking of psychiatry*. New York, NY: Scribe.

Hansard (2018). Prescription Drugs: Children: Written Question – 128871. [Online.] *Hansard*; 21 February. www.parliament.uk/business/publications/written-questions-answers-statements/written-question/Commons/2018-02-21/128871 (accessed 26 June 2019).

Harrow M, Jobe TH (2007). Factors involved in outcome and recovery in schizophrenia patients not on antipsychotic medications: a 15-year multifollow-up study. *Journal of Nervous and Mental Disease* *195*(5): 406–414.

Harrow M, Jobe TH, Faull RN (2012). Do all schizophrenia patients need antipsychotic treatment continuously throughout their lifetime? A 20-year longitudinal study. *Psychological Medicine 42*(10): 2145–2155.

Healy D (2006). Did regulators fail over selective serotonin reuptake inhibitors? *British Medical Journal 333*(7558): 92–95.

Johnson CF, Macdonald HJ, Atkinson P, Buchanan AI, Downes N, Dougall N (2012). Reviewing long-term antidepressants can reduce drug burden: a prospective observational cohort study. *British Journal of General Practice 62*(11): e773–e779.

Johnstone L (2014). *A Straight Talking Introduction to Diagnosis*. Ross-on-Wye: PCCS Books.

Kinderman P (2014). *A New Prescription for Psychiatry: why we need a whole new approach to mental health and well-being*. London: Palgrave MacMillan.

Kirk SA, Gomory T, Cohen D (2015). *Mad Science: psychiatric coercion, diagnosis, and drugs*. Piscataway, NJ: Transaction Publishers.

Kirk SA, Kutchins H (1992). *The Selling of DSM: the rhetoric of science in psychiatry*. Hawthorne: Aldine de Gruyter.

Kirmayer LJ, Minas H (2000). The future of cultural psychiatry. *Canadian Journal of Psychiatry 45*(5): 438–446.

Kitanaka J (2013) *Depression in Japan: psychiatric cures for a society in distress*. Princeton, NJ: Princeton University Press.

Kondro W, Sibbald B (2004). Drug company experts advised to withhold data about SSRI use in children. *Canadian Medical Association Journal 170*: 783.

Kutchins N, Kirk SA (1997). *Making Us Crazy: DSM: the psychiatric bible and the creation of mental disorders*. New York, NY: The Free Press.

Lacasse JR, Leo J (2005). Serotonin and depression: a disconnect between the advertisements and the scientific literature. *PLoS Med 2*(12): e392.

The Lancet (2012). Editorial: living with grief. *The Lancet 379*(9816): 589.

Ledford H (2012). Diagnostics tome comes under fire. *Nature 482*: 14–15.

Lexchin J, Bero LA, Djulbegovic B, Clark O (2003). Pharmaceutical industry sponsorship and research outcome and quality: systematic review. *British Medical Journal 326*: 1167–1170.

Lo B, Field MJ (2009). *Conflict of Interest in Medical Research, Education, and Practice*. Institute of Medicine (US) Committee on Conflict of Interest in Medical Research, Education, and Practice. Washington, DC: National Academies Press.

National Institute for Health and Care Excellence (NICE) (2009). *Depression in adults: recognition and management*. London: NICE.

NHS Digital (2017). *Prescriptions Dispensed in the Community – Statistics for England, 2006–2016*. [Online.] https://digital.nhs.uk/data-and-information/publications/statistical/prescriptions-dispensed-in-the-community/prescriptions-dispensed-in-the-community-statistics-for-england-2006-2016-pas (accessed 26 June 2019).

Orlowski JP, Wateska L (1992). The effects of pharmaceutical firm enticements on physician prescribing patterns. *Chest 102*: 270–273.

Salvo F, Pariente A, Shakir S et al (2016). Sudden cardiac and sudden unexpected death related to antipsychotics: a meta-analysis of observational studies. *Clinical Pharmacology & Therapeutics 99*: 306–314.

Schulz N (2004). Did antidepressants depress Japan? [Online.] *New York Times*: 22 August. https://www.nytimes.com/2004/08/22/magazine/did-antidepressants-depress-japan.html?pagewanted=all&src=pm (accessed 26 June 2019).

Skultans V (2003). From damaged nerves to masked depression: inevitability and hope in Latvian psychiatric narratives. *Social Science and Medicine 56*(12): 2421–2431.

Smith BL (2012). Inappropriate prescribing. Monitor on Psychology 43(6): 36. www.apa.org/monitor/2012/06/prescribing (accessed 29 July 2019).

Smith R (2005). Medical journals are an extension of the marketing arm of pharmaceutical companies. *PLoS Med 2*(5): e138.

Spielmans GI, Parry PI (2010). From evidence-based medicine to marketing-based medicine: evidence from internal industry documents. *Bioethical Inquiry 7*: 13–29.

Spurling GK, Mansfield PR, Montgomery BD et al (2010). Information from pharmaceutical companies and the quality, quantity, and cost of physicians' prescribing: a systematic review. *PLoS Medicine 7*(10): e1000352.

Timimi S (2008). Child psychiatry and its relationship with the pharmaceutical industry: theoretical and practical issues. *Advances in Psychiatric Treatment 14*: 3–9.

Turner EH, Matthews AM, Linardatos E et al (2008). Selective publication of antidepressant trials and its influence on apparent efficacy. *The New England Journal of Medicine 17*: 252–260.

Watters E (2011). *Crazy Like Us: the globalisation of the Western mind*. New York, NY: Robinson Publishing.

Whitaker R (2017). Psychiatry Under the Influence. In: Davies J (ed). *The Sedated Society: the causes and harms of our psychiatric drug epidemic*. London: Palgrave Macmillan (pp163–188).

Whitaker R (2016). *Rising Prescriptions, Rising Disability – Is There a Link?* [Video.] All-Party Parliamentary Group for Prescribed Drug Dependence event on link between rising prescribing and disability, 11 May 2016. http://cepuk.org/2016/05/27/video-now-available-appg-event-link-rising-prescribing-disability/ (accessed 26 June 2019).

Whitaker R, Cosgrove L (2015). *Psychiatry Under the Influence: institutional corruption, social injury, and prescriptions for reform*. New York, NY: Palgrave Macmillan.

World Health Organization (2018). *International Classification of Diseases (11th revision) (ICD-11)*. Geneva: WHO.

Wunderink L, Nieboer RM, Wiersma D, Sytema S, Nienhuis FJ (2013). Recovery in remitted first-episode psychosis at 7 years of follow-up of an early dose reduction/discontinuation or maintenance treatment strategy: long-term follow-up of a 2-year randomized clinical trial. *Journal of the American Medical Association 70*(9): 913–920.

7 The language of values; the value of language

Clare Shaw

For the past 15 years, I've had a dual career. As a mental health trainer, researcher and activist, I have been overtly informed by my own experiences of trauma, breakdown and mental health service use – and, specifically, the experience of being diagnosed with 'borderline personality disorder' (BPD). At the same time, I've developed a career as poet: I have three collections with Bloodaxe; I work with a wide range of organisations, including the Wordsworth Trust, the Poetry School and the Arvon Foundation, and I'm currently a Royal Literary Fellow.

These apparently distinct careers are united by language. Language is the medium in which we make sense of the world and each other. It's how we give shape to our ideas and experiences and how we communicate them to each other. As mental health practitioners, activists and survivors, language is central to our task of offering support, facilitating personal and social change and surviving difficult experiences. We aim for a language that gives a helpful shape to thoughts and experiences, enabling us to make sense of the world and ourselves in a way that matches our values and vision and facilitates effective communication.

As our primary means of constructing and sharing meaning, words can help and heal us, but they can also do terrible harm. I use the word 'table' and, without any further descriptors, you know that I mean a four-legged item of furniture with a level surface, commonly used for placing items on. It is impossible to deny the usefulness of labels; they enable us to live and move through the world, to identify our emotions, to give words to difficult experiences, and to seek solidarity with others – women, survivors, LGBTQ, for example.

However, 'BPD' does not exist in the way that a table exists. 'BPD' does not describe a biological system or set of processes such as the flu virus or osteoarthritis.

While common consensus holds that 'BPD' is caused by a combination of genetic and environmental factors, in reality, no genetic factors have been identified. And while labels like 'table' or 'blue' or 'joy' seem to be a relatively value-free way of grouping together a set of similar experiences and perceptions, many others are heavy with negative values. These labels reflect cultural attitudes and assumptions in a viscerally vicious way; they are so damaging to individuals and collectives that we physically recoil from reading or saying them.

Language can hurt

'BPD' reflects the assumption that the individual is damaged and bad. Whatever an individual has suffered – rape, abuse, homophobia, poverty – the linguistic category of 'BPD' states that the cause of their distress exists within them. The individual – rather than the traumatic experience, the family, the society – becomes the problem. Coping strategies, ingenuity, courage, the drive to survive are reframed in the language of 'disorder'.

Mental health professionals, service users and activists need to recognise language as the most important tool we have at our disposal for making meaning of the world. We need to treat it with the respect it deserves. We need a language that reflects not just our political values but also the value, complexity, intensity and inherent contradictions of all experience. We should be aware of the language we use. Language is what marks us out as truly human. Language is a gift.

The one who cannot speak, the one who is silent, the one whose words are trapped inside her – she's the one who can tell you about language. The one who has walked away from language – she understands how words work

(that words are bricks that trap you, that can build you a house with no windows you cannot see out)

(that words are pins, there no malice in them but they have you stuck)

who knows that words are gold, heavy and yellow, you pluck them from the ground like roots, messy, like heavy sunshine pouring down. Who knows what gold means, how many have died for it

The one who will not speak whose words are all inside her who runs from the words each day and by night they come pouring back into her brain the ways butterflies do or fish all in a panic, how the sky then is full of them, she cannot breathe

– she's the one who can tell you about language –

whose voice is a large fish trapped inside her, she feels it turn and flip, it has sunk to the very deep where no light is, or warmth where the pressure would crush a man, the deep eternal dark,

whose voice survives on the fallout of other creatures, small bodies.

Let her tell you. Let her begin.

What are words but balloons – empty noises? Why bother? What's a balloon unhitched from its tether?

Words never picked a girl up in a churchyard in the earliest days of July when the other kids were in the park, she was picking leaves for her rabbits; words didn't make the sun pour down like water; and the small flowers wither in the heat. Words

did not hoist her up, bodily, though she was tall for her age and substantial, words did not dress her that morning in a striped white T-shirt she would remember forever for its pushing right up to her neck, for the way it came back in a bag with dust on it; it did not smell of her anymore, she would never wear it again

did not carry her to the low steep slope and the bushes and lie her down, did not strip her

it was not words over her mouth to stop her screaming (no word could stop her from screaming)

and when nobody came, no help, that space that should have held a kind man, a strong man, someone's mother, a phone to stop it from happening,

that space was more than just words

and the police in their cars with their glances, their silence, their anywhere faces, they were not just words

and the station they took her to, and the smell of metal and piss, and the Doctor.

It was not words that undressed her on a sheet of plastic, and swabbed her, and noted the marks, the bitemarks, the grazes

the scratches from the branches where she'd laid

and the dandelions which she had to find, without them it was all just words, they wouldn't believe in the sun, how it poured through the branches above her

she couldn't believe

how easy she was to pick up; she'd never trust her weightedness again.

There they were; small, multiple, crushed, still warm, she thought, from her hand

despite the Doctor, who said that he must do this – his fingers, his swabs, the paper on the table where she lay – because girls tell lies

and she assents and never forgets this

and the statement, pages of it, the policewoman who asked her for words she wrote in an adult hand

but there were some she chose not to speak, there are some things too shameful for words

like, how when it was over, she said

out of relief at not being dead, the ingrained habit of manners

that wasn't so bad

and would never, ever forget

or forgive this

Like the time, 20 years later, when already her life was full of doctor after doctor, and strip lights, and long corridors smelling of chemicals and men

how she was punched to the floor, where she lay in the street and observed with some interest her

head snapped backwards and forwards with each kick, how the small bones bent and shattered

how she waited all day for the police who never turned up

how the manager called them for her and talked

about the alleged assault

(it did not feel alleged to her)

(or the bruises which lingered for months).

Words are not balloons, wood, are not paint. Are not even paintings. She cannot throw them away. Words leave their print like fingers or bruises. Permanent.

The words they used for her were not unhitched. Were not detached. She absorbed them. She lived them. It was words that did for her.

Or this – her T-shirt returned in its bag, and her shorts, and the shame of no knickers. And the call to her mother who would rather, through all of this, have been anywhere, anywhere else, and this she knew through every living second of it, and there were so many

The call to say he was caught, charged, pleaded guilty

Which was a good thing, because now she would not have to tell her own story, it would not be necessary to speak (aloud) her life again

and to know he pleaded guilty to indecent assault: indecent (not in keeping with accepted standards of what is right or proper in polite society).

(that sunshine pouring down on her, the morning lake, the fish, the heavy green water)

The taking of indecent liberties.

(that tall wall with its angles, the dust, the sky and no clouds, the dandelions dying in her hand)

Unacceptable behaviour –

(the twigs in her back, the grazes, the rabbits thumping and hungry in their hutches, the rumble of traffic passing)

– including but not restricted to unwanted oral sex

and yes, it was true that she was the spoiled sky. That she was the sour earth after rain, that she was the bad smell rising. That she was a baby, wounded, she would never be better again. And how this was said to her mattered.

And how this was said to her mattered.

She was a girl to whom language did matter

over and over

She was a good girl

A baby who did not cry

A girl who never asked for anything directly

a girl who always said please and thankyou

she was a girl who was handy with words and their worlds

she was a girl subject to unwanted sexual behaviour contrary to the accepted standards of polite society

who had all the words in the world and could not use them

who made of herself then a sculpture, knowing every shape, every shade has its meaning

and her meaning was all about pain

and by this I mean vomit, years of it, by this I mean

no food. By this I mean eye sockets so dry she couldn't see anything but directly in front of her, I mean the silver-white high of hunger, over, over, day after night

I mean wounds, deliberate, I mean the wide-eyed gape of a cut, I mean the brimming of blood and the hot flood of it, I mean bandages, stuck under sleeves that were not lifted

I mean the banging of the head, the taste of earth and rust; I mean the thump of a baseball bat on the wrist on the shin I mean the river the water so cold it was a stone stamped hard either side of the head

I mean pills in their thousands, the weep and the gulp, the rocking, the retching, the sleep

and no words for it but

eventually she said

help (please)

----

and how then it started in earnest

she had third year nerves (obviously)
clinical depression (untypical)
anxiety disorder (non-responsive)
bulimia nervosa (mild)
she had (query) borderline personality disorder she had
(definitely) borderline personality disorder (untreatable)
she was hopeless
she was a classic case

and the words left their bruises until she forgot her own skin, its original shade

then words did for her

words that had her locked up

words that she swallowed each morning

until

how could she find her own shape?

words had her gripped her by the ribs and twisted

words did for her

held her and told they had all the answers could set her straight could make it all alright then fucked her over and over (and not in a good way)

put her in a dark room with a shadow that smelled like a woman and a sound like choking

she could not find the bed

put her in a white room with no one to talk to

and a warm room where a man put his hand down her pants

and a sunlit room fuggy with sweat with women who talked and one who played with words like they were balloons that had no substance, words like seeds in the breeze that had nothing to do with her

but her words were heavy, they were wood, they were solid. They told her

exactly
who
she
was

----

wrong not just in the head but the centre, where it hurts, heavily, day-after-day

wrong where it counts. Told her

that she was not, and never could again be

that little creature,

and never again not sad, plainly, or happy, somewhere in between, or angry, or nothing, or so ashamed she must always dream of being someone else, or pissed off at the over-pricing in the Co-op. No, now she will be

Borderline Personality Disorder (read

untreatable, unstable, hysterical, manipulative, self-destructive. Read posturing, immature, time-wasting, gesturing, hopeless and weak. Difficult patient. Unworthy of treatment. Dishonest, dangerous, not-to-be-trusted, non-compliant, unreasonably angry and above all, seeking of attention which must by all means be denied)

Borderline Personality Disorder (read

will never be anyone's friend or lover, never safely be anyone's mother, never be doctor or writer or leader, never a holder of trust. Creative, possible, in their own (limited) (troubled) way, not articulate except by some trick of the light, nor beautiful given the mess. Read general loser, user of service and substance, client and resident, inmate, detainee, imprisoned or sectioned, disliked, damned), read

all wrong
as you were in the beginning are now and ever will be
amen

Borderline Personality Disorder (read

it was all your own fault

that afternoon

the heavy sun bowed in the branches

the hoods and the boots of the two men with blades

that traffic, her father, her face, everything

and that boy with the head full of stubble

that boy with the head full of stubble)

----

what did language ever do
for her (you tell me)

you tell me
please

8 | 'Schizophrenia' – the least scientific and most damaging of psychiatric labels

John Read and Lorenza Magliano

'Schizophrenia' does not exist. That is not to say some people don't have experiences that are unusual, difficult to understand, and distressing. What we are arguing here is that there is no such thing as a scientific construct called 'schizophrenia'.

Generally, we expect a psychiatric diagnosis to mean that the doctor making that diagnosis knows what the problem is and how to help. Psychiatric diagnoses suggest that the behaviours and feelings they seek to categorise are medical illnesses, like diabetes or pneumonia. They purport to explain the patient's behaviours and feelings: 'She is feeling depressed because she has depressive disorder,' or 'He is hearing voices because he has schizophrenia.'

We argue here that psychiatric diagnoses actually explain nothing and, moreover, often conceal the true sources of human misery and confusion. They are frequently misleading and, at worst, can be life destroying, because of the associated 'diagnostic pessimism' about outcomes and the stigma of mental illness. 'Schizophrenia' is, we argue, just a word that was invented more than 100 years ago and has damaged millions of lives since. It has also blocked scientific endeavours to understand the experiences that attract the label, such as hearing voices and feeling persecuted.

The invention of a non-existent illness

'Schizophrenia' was invented, in two stages, by Emil Kraepelin and Eugen Bleuler, the 'grandfathers' of modern psychiatry (Bentall, 2009; Read, 2013a). Throughout the 19th century, progress in medicine had been impressive, and the new discipline of psychiatry needed to catch up and demonstrate that its doctors were more than simply madhouse keepers. The profession's very survival as a medical science was at stake.

Kraepelin claimed to have discovered a group of people in whom psychological deterioration begins in adolescence and continues into dementia (Kraepelin, 1893). He called it 'dementia praecox' ('praecox' meaning 'early'). Essentially, he made a list of common behaviours and applied a medical-sounding label to them, which he claimed proved the existence of the 'illness' because, he asserted, the people who had it were exhibiting its 'symptoms'. This is circular logic.

In 1911, Eugen Bleuler coined the word 'schizophrenia' to rename Kraepelin's 'dementia praecox' (1911/1950). He abandoned the idea that all those with the symptoms ended up with 'dementia', stating: 'It is impossible to describe all the variations which the course of schizophrenia may take' (p328). He also admitted: 'We do not as yet know with certainty the primary symptoms of the schizophrenic cerebral disease' (p349) and, 'The pathology of schizophrenia gives us no indication as to where we should look for the causes of the disease' (p337) and, 'We do not know what the schizophrenic process actually is' (p466).

Kraepelin's list included no fewer than 36 groups of 'psychic' symptoms and 19 physical symptoms (1913/1919). A patient could have any of these symptoms in any combination and still get the same diagnosis as another with a completely different set. However, his attempts to find physiological evidence failed: autopsies, conducted by the famous Alois Alzheimer, revealed nothing (Bentall 2009: 31), and Kraepelin was forced to admit that the causes were 'at the present time still wrapped in impenetrable darkness' (1913/1919: 224). The key words are 'at the present time'. That 'to be proved later' clause is still used today by genetic and brain researchers still seeking a biological cause for 'schizophrenia'.

Behavioural symptoms included:

They conduct themselves in a free and easy way, and laugh on serious occasions. (Kraepelin, 1913/1919: 34)

They go about in untidy and dirty clothes, unwashed, unkempted, go with a lighted cigar into church. (Kraepelin, 1913/1919: 34)

The patients sit about idle, trouble themselves about nothing, do not go to their work. (Kraepelin, 1913/1919: 37)

Patients are in love with a ward-mate with complete disregard of sex, ugliness, or even repulsiveness. (Bleuler, 1911/1950: 52)

It hardly makes any difference to the patient whether he is addressing a person in authority or someone more humbly-placed whether a man or a woman. (Bleuler, 1911/1950: 49)

> A hebephrenic [subtype] whose very speech was confusion, held the cigar-holder to the mouth of another patient suffering from muscular atrophy… with a patience and indefatigability of which no normal person would ever be capable. (Bleuler, 1911/1950: 48)

> Perversions like homosexuality and similar anomalies are often indicated in the whole behaviour and in the dress of the patient. (Bleuler, 1924: 188)

'Flat affect' and 'inappropriate affect' (essentially, having any feelings) were regarded as 'primary symptoms'. Feeling two opposing emotions was also abnormal – 'ambivalence' being a defining characteristic of 'schizophrenia'. Remembering feelings too intensely was also a symptom: 'Even decades later… nuances of sexual pleasure, embarrassment, pain or jealously, may emerge in all their vividness which we never find in the healthy' (Bleuler, 1911/1950: 46).

'Wrong pathways of thought' carried 'the schizophrenic mark of the bizarre' (Bleuler, 1911/1950: 25). They are wrong because they are 'pathways deviating from experience' (Bleuler, 1911/1950: 354). Since a thought is necessarily part of one's experience, whose experience is it deviating from? Kraepelin (1913/1919) defined 'incoherence of thought' in terms of whether psychiatrists can understand their patients, highlighting 'that peculiarly bewildering incomprehensibility' (p20). He could have recommended that the ability to understand unusual thinking be added to psychiatric training curricula, but instead he added 'incomprehensibility' to his symptom list.

Bleuler (1911/1950: 14) found some types of thinking bewildering, noting that '[t]wo ideas fortuitously encountered, are combined into one thought' and '[t]he inclination to cling to one idea to which the patient then returns again and again'. Bringing together ideas to form new ideas is the trademark of artists and philosophers. Holding steadfastly to one belief characterises the religious or political enthusiast. Did he really intend to pathologise these groups?

> Poets and musicians must also be more sensitive than other people, a quality which is a hindrance to the daily tasks of life and often attains the significance of a disease.
> (Bleuler, 1924: 172)

> Many schizophrenics display lively affect at least in certain directions. Among them are the active writers, the world improvers, the health fanatics, the founders of new religions. (Bleuler, 1911/1950: 41)

What is left? What is considered sane? We must obey our superiors, want to work, be heterosexual, not feel too much or too little, not remember too vividly, not get too interested in new ideas, not show too much compassion, not write too much poetry or play too much music, not try to change the world, and, when distressed, we must speak in a way that even psychiatrists can understand.

Psychiatric diagnosis has been questioned since its very inception. In 1922, the textbook *Mental Diseases* concluded: 'Psychiatric diagnoses do not contribute anything of value whatever to our knowledge of symptomatology, diagnosis or treatment' (May, 1922: 246). By 1949 it had been established that: 'The psychiatric taxonomy which psychologists have been constrained to adopt is so inadequate, even for psychiatry, that no patching can fix it up' (Roe, 1949: 38). Yet it prevailed, despite consistent findings from scientific research that question the very foundations on which it rests.

Reliability: can we agree on what 'schizophrenia' is and who has it?

For a concept to exist, it has to pass a 'reliability' test. That is, it has to satisfy the key issue of whether we can agree on who has it.

As early as 1949, a study found that pairs of psychiatrists made the same diagnosis in only 33% to 50% of cases (Ash, 1949). Beck and colleagues (1962) managed to increase agreement for 'schizophrenia' to 53% (or 42%, allowing for agreement by chance) by employing artificial research conditions so as to maximise reliability. But, when 134 American and 194 British psychiatrists were given an identical case study, 69% of the Americans and only two per cent of the British gave a diagnosis of 'schizophrenia' (Copeland et al, 1971).

In the famous 'On Being Sane in Insane Places' study (Rosenhan, 1975), eight 'normal' people sought help from psychiatric services, saying they kept hearing the words 'hollow', 'empty' and 'thud'. All were admitted to psychiatric hospital and seven were diagnosed 'schizophrenic'. None of the staff realised that the pseudo-patients were 'normal', although many fellow patients did. In a follow-up study, the psychiatrists were warned to expect pseudo-patients to present for treatment; this produced a 21% detection rate – but no pseudo-patients had actually sought their help (Rosenhan, 1975). This study was partially replicated 30 years later (Slater, 2004).

As Bentall relates (2009), schizophrenia was continually redefined throughout the 20th century, most significantly, and famously, based on Schneider's 'first-rank symptoms' such as 'hallucinations' and 'delusions'. The *Diagnostic and Statistical Manual of Mental Disorders* (*DSM*), psychiatry's diagnostic bible, was first published in 1952, but has since seen multiple revisions and expansions. The 'neo-Kraepelinians' (Bentall, 2009) who were responsible for the 1980 third edition had overseen a massive research project to try to develop new definitions and 'symptom' checklists that might increase reliability. By 1987, however, the American Psychiatric Association (APA) admitted:

> Despite extensive field testing of the *DSM–III* diagnostic criteria before their official adoption, experience with them since their publication had revealed,

> as expected, many instances in which the criteria were not entirely clear,
> were inconsistent across categories, or were even contradictory. (APA, 1987)

Fifty years ago, British psychologist Don Bannister had recommended that 'research into schizophrenia as such, should not be undertaken':

> Schizophrenia as a concept, is a semantic Titanic, doomed before it sails, a
> concept so diffuse as to be unusable in a scientific context… We diagnose
> one person as schizophrenic because he manifests characteristics A and
> B and diagnose a second person as schizophrenic because he manifests
> characteristics C, D and E. The two people are now firmly grouped
> in the same category while not specifically possessing any common
> characteristic… Disjunctive categories are logically too primitive for
> scientific use. (Bannister, 1968: 181)

In 1992, after a lifetime studying diagnoses, psychiatrist Ian Brockington concluded:

> It is important to loosen the grip which the concept of 'schizophrenia' has
> on the minds of psychiatrists. Schizophrenia is an idea whose very essence
> is equivocal, a nosological category without natural boundaries, a barren
> hypothesis. Such a blurred concept is not a valid object of scientific enquiry.
> (Brockington 1992: 207)

Brockington decried 'a babble of precise but different formulations of the same concept'. In the same year, researchers identified 16 systems for classifying 'schizophrenia'. In a study of 248 patients 'designed to maximise reliability and agreement' (Herron, Schultz & Welt, 1992), the number diagnosed as 'schizophrenic' by these 16 systems ranged from one to 203.

Today, to receive a diagnosis of schizophrenia using the most recent edition, *DSM-5* (APA, 2013), you need two out of five 'characteristic symptoms': 'hallucinations', 'delusions', 'disorganised speech', 'disorganised or catatonic behaviour' and 'negative symptoms'. There are still multiple ways (1 + 2 vs 3 + 4; 1 + 2 vs 3 + 5 etc) in which two people can meet the criteria without sharing any symptoms. The scientific term for this, as applied by Bannister above, is 'disjunctive'. In ordinary language, the correct term, if one wished to be polite, would be 'nonsense'.

The World Health Organization has produced an alternative diagnostic system, the *International Classification of Diseases* (*ICD*), now in its 11th revision (World Health Organization, 2018). This is even more problematic than the *DSM*. It doesn't include the *DSM* requirement that 'continuous signs of the disturbance persist for at least six months'; instead, it requires only one month. You can even be diagnosed with 'schizophrenia, in full remission' when you no longer have any 'symptoms' at all, thereby reinforcing the cruel notion that no one ever really recovers from this 'illness'.

So the construct is still disjunctive and, therefore, scientifically meaningless. It should have been discarded decades ago. Indeed, Dr Christian Fibiger, a former vice-president of neuroscience at the drug industrial giant Eli Lilly, has predicted that 'concepts such as schizophrenia will surely be discarded and future generations will look back and might rightfully ask "What were they thinking?"' (Fibiger, 2012: 50).

Validity: is 'schizophrenia' what it is supposed to be?

Even when reliability *is* demonstrated, that does not guarantee validity. Nearly 50 years ago, two expert diagnosticians wrote:

> Class membership conveys little information beyond the gross symptomatology of the patient and contributes little to the solution of the pressing problems of aetiology, treatment procedures, prognosis, etc. (Zigler & Phillips, 1961: 612)

Furthermore, investigating validity is meaningless without reliability. If we can't agree on who has 'schizophrenia' – if the 'schizophrenics' one researcher studies differ from those studied by other researchers – then its properties cannot be evaluated.

If reliability *had* been established, however, we would then investigate whether the construct is related to things that the theory underpinning the construct claims it is related to. In the case of 'mental illnesses', we would look for a) a set of symptoms that occur together but not in other 'mental illnesses'; b) a predictable outcome, c) a biological cause, and d) a positive response to medical treatments.

Symptoms

There is no evidence of a set of 'schizophrenic' behaviours and experiences that occur together but do not occur in other conditions. In 1973, the World Health Organization compared clusters of symptoms that occur together in real people with the groupings produced by diagnostic categories. It was found that 'Patients diagnosed as schizophrenic are distributed in all clusters. No single "schizophrenic profile" was elicited' (WHO, 1973: 350).

'Schizophrenic' symptoms are frequently found in people with other 'disorders'. Conversely, most people diagnosed 'schizophrenic' have sufficient symptoms of other 'disorders' to earn additional diagnoses. This 'co-morbidity' has been found in relation to 'depression', 'obsessive-compulsive disorder', 'panic disorder', 'dissociative disorders', 'bipolar disorder', 'personality disorders', 'substance abuse', 'post-traumatic stress disorder' and 'anxiety disorders' (Crow, 2010; Read, 2013b).

Outcomes

There is no evidence that people given the 'schizophrenia' diagnosis have a common outcome. Three findings characterise long-term studies: a) massive variations in outcomes, b) many people labelled 'schizophrenic' recover, c) the best predictors are psychosocial factors (Read, 2013b).

Estimates of long-term recovery rates vary from 13% to 72%, with most falling between 30% and 55% (Read, 2013b). Ciompi (1980: 42) concluded:

> What is called 'the course of schizophrenia' more closely resembles a life process open to a great variety of influences of all kinds than an illness with a given course.

After a century of pessimism during which this diagnosis had damaged the lives of millions, a review by the WHO International Study of Schizophrenia (ISoS) proclaimed:

> The ISoS joins others in relieving patients, carers and clinicians of the chronicity paradigm which dominated thinking throughout much of the 20th century. (Harrison et al, 2001: 513)

Thus the diagnosis 'schizophrenia' has no predictive validity. Furthermore, the huge variability in outcome is best predicted by psychosocial factors (Read, 2103b). Predictors of poor outcome include adverse life events; poor social or cognitive skills; poor academic or work performance; high involvement with over-involved, critical families; being unmarried (especially in men); high anxiety; substance abuse (Read, 2013b; Harrison et al, 2001), and defining oneself as 'mentally ill' (Yanos, Roe & Lysaker, 2010).

One final example of inconsistent outcomes and psychosocial factors predicting outcome is the fact that outcomes from 'schizophrenia' in poorer countries are far superior to those in wealthy, industrialised societies (Harrison et al, 2001).

Biological causes

For the past few decades, three 'facts' have been repeatedly presented in textbooks, on drug company websites and in their 'educational' pamphlets to show that 'schizophrenia' is a biologically based illness:

1. 'Schizophrenia' occurs with equal frequency in all countries.
2. The brains of 'schizophrenics' are abnormal.
3. There is a genetic predisposition to 'schizophrenia'.

The first of the three 'proofs' that schizophrenia is a medical illness is that it occurs in the same proportion (about one per cent) internationally. This is supposed to prove that environmental factors are irrelevant, and the cause must therefore be biological. However, many real medical illnesses show huge variations between populations and locations. Furthermore the 'facts' on which this silly idea was based are not true (Read, 2013c). Thirty years ago, an international review of more than 70 prevalence studies had already reported that the highest rate was 55 times greater than the lowest (Torrey, 1987).

A more sensible way to try to prove that 'schizophrenia' is a medical illness is to show that 'schizophrenic' and 'normal' brains differ. However, there are three important issues that are ignored when drawing conclusions about causation from brain research. The first is the lack of reliability of the construct under investigation. Second, if 'schizophrenic' brains are different, it does not mean we have found the cause of the 'symptoms'. When we are grieving the loss of a loved one, our brains act differently from usual. Is our sadness caused by the brain's slower functioning or by our loss? Most studies of the brains of 'schizophrenics' ignore external events. It is as if psychiatric brain researchers fail to grasp that the brain is designed to respond to the environment. What use would a brain be if that were not so (Read et al, 2014)?

The third ignored issue is that one of the external events that can negatively alter the brains of 'schizophrenics' is antipsychotic medication (Ho et al, 2011; Hutton et al, 2013).

Biochemistry

The term 'chemical imbalance' is promoted as an explanation for many 'mental health problems' (Read & Sanders, 2010). Biological psychiatry's lead theory of 'schizophrenia' is that it is caused by too much dopamine. Antipsychotic drugs, originally used for pre-surgery sedation, were first used on 'schizophrenics' in the 1950s. It was only discovered later that one of their many effects was to block dopamine receptors. Psychiatry jumped to the conclusion that, if these drugs cure 'schizophrenia' *and* block the dopamine system, then the cause of 'schizophrenia' must be over-activity of the dopamine system. This is as sensible as arguing that headaches are caused by lack of aspirin (Jackson, 1986).

The drugs not only block the dopamine system, they also initiate an attempt by the brain to compensate for the blockage (Hutton et al, 2013). So, over-activity in the dopamine system can be caused by the drugs that are supposedly treating the 'illness' that is supposed to be caused by over-activity in the dopamine system.

Brain anatomy

Another key component of the quest to prove 'schizophrenia' is a medical illness is the finding that some 'schizophrenics' have large spaces in their brains. The enlargement of these fluid-filled gaps, called ventricles, is related to reduction (atrophy) in brain tissue, particularly in the frontal cortex. As Richard Bentall points out (2009: 153): 'For many biological psychiatrists, this has been taken as incontestable evidence of a disease process at work', despite the three major problems with this kind of research noted above. Enlarged ventricles are found in many other disorders, including depression and alcoholism, so are not a specific cause of 'schizophrenia'. All we know is that some people labelled 'schizophrenic' have experienced some of the factors that cause enlarged ventricles, such as trauma, excessive alcohol and – again – psychiatric drugs. A large MRI study found that a major cause of atrophy in the prefrontal cortex is antipsychotic medication (Ho et al, 2011).

Genetics

Space does not permit coverage of all the critiques of the woeful methodology and blatantly biased conceptualisations that led to the longstanding myth that there is a genetic basis to something called 'schizophrenia' (Bentall, 2009; Joseph, 2013, 2017). One of the most systematic and prolific of these critics concluded:

> Psychiatry's uncritical acceptance of the conclusions of schizophrenia twin and adoption researchers is an appalling development in the history of scientific research. It can be understood much more by psychiatry's interest in maintaining itself as a viable profession than on the basis of a careful analysis of the original studies. Moreover, genetic theories aid the interests of the social and political elites, and the interests of the psychopharmaceutical industry, by locating the causes of psychological distress within people's bodies and brains, as opposed to their familial, social, and political environments... Focusing attention on genetic research, regardless of the massive flaws, biases and untenable assumptions contained therein, successfully diverts attention from the social factors that contribute to people exhibiting behaviors given the schizophrenia label. (Joseph, 2013: 85)

The evidence for these social factors is far more robust than the studies the biological psychiatrists refer to when promulgating their illness notion. They include poverty, child abuse and neglect and other adversities (Longden & Read, 2016; Varese et al, 2012). For example, poverty is even more predictive of being diagnosed with 'schizophrenia' than being diagnosed with other mental health problems (Read, 2010; Read, Johnstone & Taitimu, 2013). People who were abused or neglected as a child are several times more likely to experience psychosis later in life than those who were not abused or neglected (Varese et al, 2012; Read, 2013d; Read et al, 2014). Other predictive factors include bullying, discrimination, witnessing domestic violence, prenatal stress, war trauma, torture, adulthood rape and physical assault, excessive marijuana use in adolescence, and disturbed attachment relationships with one's caregivers, including abandonment, being the result of an unwanted pregnancy, being adopted or fostered, being raised in institutional care, dysfunctional parenting (often intergenerational), and parental death or separation (Longden & Read, 2016; Varese et al, 2012).

Medical treatments

Electroshock treatment was invented to treat 'schizophrenia'. There has never been any evidence that it is more effective than placebo (Read et al, 2013). Antipsychotic drugs, while undoubtedly very powerful tranquillisers, have never been effective at curing an illness called 'schizophrenia' and have performed no more successfully than placebo at significantly reducing its supposed 'symptoms' for most users of the drugs (Bola, Kao & Soydan, 2011; Hutton et al, 2013). Moreover, there is no evidence that the long-lasting injections that have recently become prevalent are any more effective than the pills (Hutton et al, 2013). These drugs also cause a range of serious adverse effects, including severe weight gain, loss of libido, diabetes, cardiovascular disease, decreased brain volume and shortened life span (Ho et al, 2011; Hutton et al, 2013; Weinmann, Read & Aderhold, 2009).

Cochrane reviews are regarded as the most thorough and objective approach to evaluating treatments. A 2010 Cochrane review of risperidone, a commonly used antipsychotic, concluded:

> Risperidone appears to have a marginal benefit in terms of clinical improvement compared with placebo in the first few weeks of treatment but the margin may not be clinically meaningful. Global effects suggest that there is no clear difference between risperidone and placebo… People with schizophrenia or their advocates may want to lobby regulatory authorities to insist on better studies being available before wide release of a compound with the subsequent beguiling advertising. (Rattehalli, Jayaram & Smith, 2010: 18)

To again quote Christian Fibiger, a former vice-president of Eli Lilly:

> Given that there cannot be a coherent biology for syndromes as heterogeneous as schizophrenia, it is not surprising that the field has failed to validate distinct molecular targets for the purpose of developing mechanistically novel therapeutics… Psychopharmacology is in crisis. The data are in, and it is clear that a massive experiment has failed. (Fibiger 2012: 69)

Conclusion about validity

Thirty years ago, a review of the research in these four areas (symptoms, outcomes, causes and treatments) concluded that none of the four variables that are supposed to be related to 'schizophrenia' are actually related to it. '"Schizophrenia" is not a useful scientific category and that for all these years researchers have been pursuing "a ghost within the body of psychiatry"' (Bentall, Jackson & Pilgrim, 1988: 318). Nothing has changed since then; no new evidence has emerged. This has not, however, deterred psychiatry from carrying on as usual, right up to the present day. The beliefs that there *is* a thing called 'schizophrenia' and that it is a medical illness are for some psychiatrists more powerful than all the evidence that their beliefs are incorrect.

How the 'schizophrenia' label fuels prejudice and discrimination

Of all the psychosocial causes of the distress experienced by people diagnosed 'schizophrenic', one of the most damaging is discrimination. Many feel it is more disturbing than psychosis itself (Schulze et al, 2003). It is a barrier to recovery (Corrigan & Kosyluk, 2013) and a predictor of national suicide rates (Schomerus et al, 2015).

The stereotype of the 'schizophrenic', the toxic combination of dangerousness, unpredictability and not being responsible for one's own actions, is consistent over place and time (Read, Haslam & Magliano, 2013). Discrimination when seeking work, housing or insurance and rejection by friends and families are common (Read et al, 2006; Thornicroft et al, 2009). Prejudice is fuelled by the media, not only via sensationalist attributions of violence to 'schizophrenics' (Aoki et al, 2016; Cain et al, 2013) but also by the metaphorical use of the word 'schizophrenic' to denigrate people as unpredictable and irrational (Magliano, Read & Marassi, 2011; Magliano & Marassi, 2018).

Prejudice also exists among some health (Magliano et al, 2017a, 2017b) and mental health staff (Magliano, Read & Affuso, 2017). In studies of Italian GPs (Magliano et al, 2017b) and mental health staff (Magliano, Read & Affuso, 2017), 91% and 78% respectively believed that people with 'schizophrenia' are dangerous.

Discrimination, anticipated discrimination (Angermeyer et al, 2004; Thornicroft et al, 2009) and internalised stigma (Dinos et al, 2004), lead to decreased self-esteem and increased alcohol use and suicidality (Read et al, 2006). A study of 732 people diagnosed with 'schizophrenia' from 27 countries found that 64% had stopped themselves from applying for work, training or education, and 58% from looking for a close relationship, because of anticipated stigma (Ucok et al, 2012).

Such discrimination, misinformation and prejudice are fuelled by diagnostic labelling.

A 2013 review (Read, Haslam & Magliano, 2013) found that, in 28 of 31 studies (90%), bio-genetic causal beliefs were related to negative attitudes, and in 24 of 26 studies (92%), psychosocial beliefs were related to positive attitudes. Subsequently, studies of Italian medical and psychology students have found associations between belief in genetic causes and higher skepticism about psychotherapies and about possibility of recovery (Magliano et al, 2016). A 2015 review concluded:

> Although biogenetic explanations may soften public stigma by diminishing blame, they increase it by inducing pessimism, avoidance, and the belief that affected people are dangerous and unpredictable. These explanations may also induce pessimism and helplessness among affected people and reduce the empathy their treating clinicians feel for them. (Haslam & Kvaale, 2015: 399)

Another review, by the most prolific research team in this field, found that:

> Generally, biogenetic causal attributions were not associated with more tolerant attitudes; they were related to stronger rejection in most studies examining schizophrenia. (Angermeyer et al, 2011: 367)

A recent review of studies of people who themselves experience psychosis concluded that:

> Those endorsing a biogenetic model may experience higher levels of implicit stigma as well as hold more stigmatizing attitudes toward others with schizophrenia. (Carter et al, 2017: 332)

The role of the drug companies in all this is evidenced by a study showing that more than half of websites about 'schizophrenia' are funded by drug companies and that industry-sponsored sites are more likely than other sites to portray 'schizophrenia' as a debilitating, biologically based illness (Read, 2008). Meanwhile, patients who, like the public, insist that their problems have resulted from adverse life events (Carter et al, 2017; Read et al, 2006; Read, Magliano & Beavan, 2013) are told they are lacking 'insight' into the fact that they have an 'illness'. A drug company-sponsored American psychiatrist has gone so far as to claim that this 'lack of insight' – which he has tried to turn into a medical phenomenon by calling it 'anosognosia' – is 'a symptom of the illness' that people without 'insight' do not believe they have (Amador, 2010). He has even claimed to know which bit of the brain makes us disagree with biological psychiatrists.

Thus, patients and the public are taught to accept diagnostic labels by the very institutions that stand to profit from developing medications designed to treat conditions that do not, medically, exist.

Diagnostic labelling and negative attitudes

Labelling does increase belief in bio-genetic causes (Angermeyer, Holzinger &

Matschinger, 2009; Magliano et al, 2017a; Read, Magliano, Beavan, 2013). It also accomplishes another of the goals of illness-based destigmatisation programmes – endorsement of psychiatrists and their drugs (Angermeyer, Holzinger & Matschinger, 2009). In terms of stigma, however, labelling is just as damaging as the bio-genetic causal beliefs that are implied by these medical-sounding labels. Studies show that diagnostic labelling is related to:

- perceived dangerousness (Angermeyer et al, 2004; Kingdon et al, 2008; Martinez et al, 2011; Magliano et al, 2017a)

- perceived unpredictability (Kingdon et al, 2008)

- perceived lack of responsibility for own actions (Penn & Nowlin-Drummond, 2001)

- perceived lack of 'humanity' (Martinez et al, 2011)

- perceived severity of the problem (Cormack & Furnham, 1998)

- perceived dependency (Angermeyer et al, 2004)

- pessimism about recovery (Kingdon et al, 2008; Magliano et al, 2017a)

- fear (Angermeyer & Matschinger, 2003)

- rejection and desire for distance (Angermeyer et al, 2004; Angermeyer, Holzinger & Matschinger, 2009; Magliano et al, 2017a).

Labelling also affects professionals. In a study of 166 Scottish GPs, participants were asked to read cases that were identical, apart from mention of a previous diagnosis of 'schizophrenia', 'depression', 'diabetes' or no 'illness'. Those responding to the vignette mentioning 'schizophrenia' were more concerned about violence and less willing to treat the person (Lawrie, Martin & McNeill, 1998). In a study of 387 Italian GPs, the 'schizophrenia' label was associated with a biological and pessimistic view of the disorder and with perceptions of dangerousness (Magliano et al, 2017a).

This relationship between labelling and negative attitudes is also found in people who experience psychosis. A British study found that 'patients who accepted their diagnosis reported a lower perceived control over illness' and that 'depression' in 'psychotic patients' is 'linked to patients' perception of controllability of their illness and absorption of cultural stereotypes of mental illness' (Birchwood et al, 1993: 387). A survey of some 500 people in the UK diagnosed 'schizophrenic' found that more than 80% believed the diagnosis was 'damaging and dangerous' (Thomas et al, 2013).

One model that helps explain why psychiatric diagnostic labels and the bio-genetic beliefs that accompany them fuel fear, prejudice and discrimination is 'psychological essentialism'. This is the mind-set that sees social groups as having fixed, underlying essences that define who they are (Haslam & Kvaale, 2015). The strongest predictor of low discrimination is contact with the people who are the object of the discrimination (Angermeyer et al, 2004; Read & Law, 1999; Schulze et al, 2003). So, people who know of someone with a diagnosis of 'schizophrenia' are less likely to label them with presumed behaviours and symptoms. It seems sad, therefore, that this goal of the illness-model approach to increase confidence in medical professionals and treatments seems to reduce confidence in the helping capacities of the public (Riedel-Heller, Matschinger & Angermeyer, 2005), thereby reducing precisely the sort of contact needed to combat prejudice.

Alternatives to 'schizophrenia'

Just say no

Regardless of one's preferred alternative to 'schizophrenia', the first step is to just stop using such an unscientific, damaging term. This is already happening in several countries (Yamaguchi et al, 2017). In 2002, the UK's Schizophrenia Fellowship changed its name to Rethink Mental Illness. In the same year, the Japanese Society of Psychiatry and Neurology abandoned the term *Seishin Bunretsu Byo* ('mind-split-disease'), which, like 'schizophrenia', implied an untreatable, irreversible biological 'illness' that made people violent, and adopted instead *Togo Shitcho Sho* ('integration disorder'). A review of 4,677 media articles found that links to violence significantly decreased after the name change (Aoki et al, 2016). In 2012, members of the International Society for the Psychological Treatments of Schizophrenia voted to remove 'schizophrenia' from its name and became the International Society for Psychological and Social Approaches to Psychosis.

A recent review of studies on renaming 'schizophrenia' have concluded that doing so reduces stigma (Lasalvia et al, 2015; Yamaguchi et al, 2017) and facilitates communication between clinicians, users and families (Lasalvia et al, 2015). For example, the term 'psychosis', which is by no means free from stigma, is less associated with negative messages in the media than 'schizophrenia' and is more associated with psychosocial causes and solutions (Magliano & Marassi, 2018). A recent study found that if a description of someone was labeled 'schizophrenia', people had more negative attitudes to it than if it was labeled 'psychosis' (Magliano et al, 2018).

Focusing on life history and needs

The second step is to stop focusing so much on the questions 'What is wrong with you?' and 'What label should I use?' and start asking, 'What happened to you?' and 'What do you need'?

The first question tends to lead to trauma-informed services (Brooker et al, 2016; Sweeney et al, 2016). Many of our current services seem to be trauma avoidant. Two recent reviews show that most abuse and neglect are undetected by psychiatric services (Read et al, 2018a) and that what *is* disclosed to staff is usually ignored (Read et al, 2018b). A *comprehensive* life history can be used to make sense of current difficulties, using psychological formulations (Johnstone, 2014; Read & Sanders, 2010) or the new Power Threat Meaning Framework (Johnstone & Boyle, 2018), or, perhaps, common sense. The prerequisites for trauma-informed mental health services can be summarised as:

> Polices should be designed not only to mandate training but to create a positive, trauma-focused culture for the service as a whole. Without such a culture, any specific gains from forms, policies, and trainings could be short lived. The idea is that all staff engage with people in such a way that facilitates recovery from any trauma or adversity that has led to the problems that they present with, that acknowledges that different traumas and adversities might require different responses, and that, at the very least, avoids retraumatizing through practices that either reproduce the trauma with the use of force or that dismiss the occurrence or impact of abuse.
> (Read et al, 2018a)

The second question, 'What do you need?', demands at least as much attention. In our quest for the right label, we often forget to ask the most obvious of all questions: 'How can I help you?' We assume that we know better about a person's needs than the person themselves, which is extraordinarily arrogant. And we sometimes believe that a diagnostic label can inform us about a person's needs, which is just plain silly. Beyond just asking the question, quality of life measures might be useful as they cover domains such as self-esteem, relationships, housing, income, empowerment, physical health and emotional life. When the people with the 'schizophrenia' diagnosis are asked about their recovery goals, they look far beyond 'symptom' reduction (Pitt, Kilbride & Welford, 2007), focusing more on the quality of their social lives (Byrne, Davies & Morrison, 2010). A questionnaire developed with service users has 'intrapersonal' and 'interpersonal' items. Unlike 'schizophrenia', it has good reliability and validity (Neil et al, 2009), and is useful.

Reliable, meaningful constructs

Categorising is an inevitable human propensity; it is wired into our brains. If we must have names and categories, there are scientific and productive ways to categorise 'madness' without using heterogeneous, disjunctive, meaningless words. The task is to find categories about which we can agree (reliable) and that are meaningful and useful (valid). This is not difficult. The first evidence-based division was into 'positive' symptoms (additions to 'normal' experience, such as 'hallucinations' and 'delusions') and 'negative' symptoms (perceived deficits, such as 'blunted affect' and 'social withdrawal') (Andreasen & Olson, 1982). More recently it has been proposed that 'schizophrenia' be replaced with four subgroups derived from clinical experience and psychosocial research: 'sensitivity psychosis', 'drug-related psychosis', 'anxiety psychosis', and 'traumatic psychosis' (Kingdon et al, 2008) – all of which were more acceptable to people experiencing psychosis than 'schizophrenia'. Others have tried to break down the relationship between trauma and psychosis (Varese et al, 2012) into four subcategories: 'traumatic psychosis', 'neurodevelopmental psychosis', 'psychotic PTSD' and 'psychosis-induced PTSD' (Stevens, Spencer & Turkington, 2017).

Besides these valuable efforts to discover meaningful, reliable groupings of behaviours and experiences, there is an increasing focus on specific behaviours and experiences. Once we forget about the non-existent ghost of 'schizophrenia' and focus instead on definable and measurable constructs, like 'hallucinations' and 'delusions', progress is made in understanding and helping (Bentall, 2009). Constructs like 'hallucinations' and 'delusions' can be further subdivided into reliable dimensional variables such as duration, intensity, frequency, conviction and distress (Morrison, 2013).

Dimensions

Besides using only reliable variables, a second important principle is to think in terms of dimensions rather than categories. Ordinary human behaviours, thoughts and feelings vary over time and between differing social contexts. So do behaviours considered 'abnormal' (Pilgrim, 2000). A review of studies comparing dimensional and categorical representations of behaviours considered indicative of 'schizophrenia' concluded that the dimensional approach is more useful in terms of yielding information on patients' needs and outcomes (van Os & Verdoux, 2003). This dimensional approach is also helpful in showing that many of the 'normal' population have 'psychotic' experiences (Johns & van Os, 2001).

Combining the specific/reliable/measurable and the dimensional approaches produces descriptions of real people engaging in certain behaviours, thoughts or feelings to various extents at various times, depending largely on what is happening around us.

Conclusion

None of this research impacts on biological psychiatry. This demonstrates that it is not an evidence-based endeavour, or a scientific discipline. It operates more like a cult, ignoring or denigrating everything and anyone that threatens its core ideology. Far from ceasing to use their discredited bio-genetic causal hypotheses and destructive labels, industrialised countries are currently trying to export them to 'developing' countries to improve their 'mental health literacy' and encourage use of labels and drugs, under the banner of the 'Global Mental Health' movement (Fernando, 2014; Read, Haslam & Magliano, 2013). They are eagerly supported by the pharmaceutical industry in this blatantly racist, imperialist enterprise.

Understanding why such a state of affairs exists requires an understanding of the social, political and economic functions of biological psychiatry's powerfully simplistic bio-genetic ideology (Boyle, 2013; Read & Dillon, 2013), and the domination of the profession by drug companies (Whitaker, 2010).

Change will have to come from the rest of us, starting with just refusing to label one another in this meaningless and hurtful way. Just say no.

Acknowledgement

This chapter is based, with permission from Routledge, on several chapters in *Models of Madness: psychological, social and biological approaches to psychosis* (Routledge, 2013), specifically: Read, 2013a, 2013b, 2013c, 2013d; Read, Magliano & Beavan, 2013; Read, Haslam & Magliano, 2013).

References

American Psychiatric Association (APA) (2013). *Diagnostic and Statistical Manual of Mental Disorders* (5th ed). Washington, DC: APA.

American Psychiatric Association (APA) (1987). *Diagnostic and Statistical Manual of Mental Disorders* (3rd ed). Washington, DC: APA.

Amador X (2010). Poor insight in schizophrenia. *Psychiatria Hungarica 25*: 5–7.

Andreasen N, Olsen S (1982). Negative v positive schizophrenia. *Archives of General Psychiatry 39*: 789–794.

Angermeyer M, Beck M, Dietrich S, Hozinger A (2004). The stigma of mental illness: patients' anticipations and experiences. *International Journal of Social Psychiatry 50*: 153–162.

Angermeyer M, Holzinger A, Carta M, Schomerus G (2011). Biogenetic explanations and public acceptance of mental illness. *British Journal of Psychiatry 199*: 367–372.

Angermeyer M, Holzinger A, Matschinger H (2009). Mental health literacy and attitude towards people with mental illness. *European Psychiatry 24*: 225–232.

Angermeyer M, Matschinger H (2003). Public beliefs about schizophrenia and depression. *Social Psychiatry and Psychiatric Epidemiology 38*: 526–534.

Aoki A, Aoki Y, Goulden R, Kasai K, Thornicroft G, Henderson C (2016). Change in newspaper coverage of schizophrenia in Japan over 20-year period. *Schizophrenia Research 175*: 193–197.

Ash P (1949). The reliability of psychiatric diagnoses. *Journal of Abnormal and Social Psychology 4*: 272–277.

Bannister D (1968). The logical requirements of research into schizophrenia. *British Journal of Psychiatry 114*: 181–188.

Beck A, Ward C, Mendelson M (1962). Reliability of psychiatric diagnoses. *American Journal of Psychiatry 119*: 351–357.

Bentall RP (2009). *Doctoring the Mind*. London: Allen Lane.

Bentall RP, Jackson H, Pilgrim D (1988). Abandoning the concept of 'schizophrenia': some implications of validity arguments for psychological research into psychotic phenomena. *British Journal of Clinical Psychology 27*: 303–324.

Birchwood M, Mason R, MacMillan F, Healy J (1993). Depression, demoralisation and control over psychotic illness: a comparison of depressed and non-depressed patients with a chronic psychosis. *Psychological Medicine 23*: 387–395.

Bleuler E (1911/1950). *Dementia Praecox or the Group of Schizophrenias*. Zinkin J (trans). New York, NY: International Universities Press.

Bleuler E (1924). *Textbook of Psychiatry* (A Brill trans). New York: Macmillan.

Bola J, Kao D, Soydan H (2011). Antipsychotic medication for early episode schizophrenia. *Cochrane Database Systematic Review* 15 June. CD006374.

Boyle M (2013). The persistence of medicalisation. In: Coles S, Keenan S, Diamond B (eds). *Madness Contested: power and practice*. Ross-on-Wye: PCCS Books (pp3–22).

Brockington I (1992). Schizophrenia: yesterday's concept. *European Psychiatry 7*: 203–207.

Brooker C, Tocque K, Kennedy A, Brown M (2016). The care programme approach: sexual violence and clinical practice in mental health. *Journal of Forensic and Legal Medicine 43*: 97–101.

Byrne R, Davies L, Morrison A (2010). Priorities and preferences for the outcomes of treatment of psychosis: a service user perspective. *Psychosis: Psychological, Social and Integrative Approaches 2*: 210–217.

Cain B, Currie R, Danks E, Du F, Hodgson E, May J, et al (2013). 'Schizophrenia' in the Australian print and online news media. *Psychosis: Psychological, Social and Integrative Approaches 6*: 97–106.

Carter L, Read J, Pyle M, Morrison A (2017). The impact of causal explanations on outcome in people experiencing psychosis: a systematic review. *Clinical Psychology & Psychotherapy 24*: 332–347.

Ciompi L (1980). The natural history of schizophrenia in the long term. *British Journal of Psychiatry 136*: 413–420.

Copeland J, Cooper J, Kendell R, Gourlay A (1971). Differences in usage of diagnostic labels amongst psychiatrists in the British Isles. *British Journal of Psychiatry 118*: 629–640.

Cormack S, Furnham A (1998). Psychiatric labelling, sex role stereotypes and beliefs about the mentally ill. *International Journal of Social Psychiatry 44*: 235–247.

Corrigan P, Kosyluk K (2013). Erasing the stigma. *Basic and Applied Social Psychology 35*: 131–140.

Crow T (2010). The continuum of psychosis: 1986–2010. *Psychiatric Annals 40*: 115–119.

Dinos S, Stevens S, Serfaty M, Weich S, King M (2004). Stigma: the feelings and experiences of 46 people with mental illness. *British Journal of Psychiatry 184*: 176–181.

Fernando S (2014). *Mental Health Worldwide: culture, globalization and development*. Basingstoke: Palgrave Macmillan.

Fibiger H (2012). Psychiatry, the pharmaceutical industry, and the road to better therapeutics. *Schizophrenia Bulletin 38*: 649–650.

Harrison G, Hopper, K, Craig T, Laska E, Siegel C, Wanderling J et al (2001). Recovery from psychotic illness: a 15- and 25-year international follow up study. *British Journal of Psychiatry 178*: 506–517.

Haslam N, Kvaale E (2015). Biogenetic explanations of mental disorder: the mixed-blessings model. *Current Directions in Psychological Science 24*: 399–404.

Herron W, Schultz C, Welt A (1992). A comparison of 16 systems to diagnose schizophrenia. *Journal of Clinical Psychology 48*: 711–721.

Ho B, Andreasen C, Ziebell S, Pierson R, Magnotta V (2011). Long-term antipsychotic treatment and brain volumes. *Archives of General Psychiatry 68*: 128–137.

Hutton P, Weinmann S, Bola J, Read J (2013). Antipsychotic drugs. In: Read J, Dillon J (eds). *Models of Madness* (2nd ed). London: Routledge (pp105–124).

Jackson H (1986). Is there a schizotoxin? In: Eisenberg N, Glasgow D (eds). *Current Issues in Clinical Psychology*. Aldershot: Gower (pp82–101).

Johns L, van Os J (2001). The continuity of psychotic experiences in the general population. *Clinical Psychology Review 21*: 1125–1141.

Johnstone L (2014). *A Straight Talking Introduction to Psychiatric Diagnoses*. Ross-on-Wye: PCCS Books.

Johnstone L, Boyle M, with Cromby J, Dillon J, Harper D, Kinderman P, Longden E, Pilgrim D, Read J (2018). *The Power Threat Meaning Framework: towards the identification of patterns in emotional distress, unusual experiences and troubled or troubling behaviour, as an alternative to functional psychiatric diagnosis*. Leicester: British Psychological Society.

Joseph J (2017). *Schizophrenia and Genetics: the end of an illusion*. E-book. Bookbaby.

Joseph J (2013). 'Schizophrenia' and heredity: Why the emperor (still) has no genes. In: Read J, Dillon J (eds). *Models of Madness* (2nd ed). London: Routledge (pp72–89).

Kingdon D, Gibson A, Kinoshita Y, Turkington D, Rathod S, Morrison A (2008). Acceptable terminology and subgroups in schizophrenia. *Social Psychiatry and Psychiatric Epidemiology 43*: 239–243.

Kraepelin E (1913/1919). Dementia praecox. In *Psychiatrica* (8th ed) (Barclay R, trans). Melbourne, FL: Krieger.

Kraepelin E (1893). *Psychiatrie* (4th ed). Leipzig: Barth.

Lasalvia A, Penta E, Sartorius N, Henderson S (2015). Should the label 'schizophrenia' be abandoned? *Schizophrenia Research 162*: 276–284.

Lawrie S, Martin K, McNeill G (1998). General practitioners' attitudes to psychiatric and medical illness. *Psychological Medicine 28*: 1463–1467.

Longden E, Read J (2016). Social adversity in the etiology of psychosis: a review of the evidence. *American Journal of Psychotherapy 70*: 5–33.

Magliano L, Marassi R (2018). 'Schizophrenia' and 'psychosis' in Italian national newspapers: do these terms convey different messages? *Schizophrenia Research*; 19 February. doi: 10.1016/j.schres.2018.02.021

Magliano L, Read J, Affuso G (2017). Predictors of staff attitudes toward schizophrenia treatments. *Psychiatric Services 68*: 1321.

Magliano L, Read J, Marassi R (2011). Metaphoric and non-metaphoric use of the term 'schizophrenia' in Italian newspapers. *Social Psychiatry and Psychiatric Epidemiology 46*: 1019–1025.

Magliano L, Petrillo M, Ruggiero G, Schioppa G (2018). Schizophrenia and psychosis: does changing the label change the beliefs? *Schizophrenia Research 193*: 482–483.

Magliano L, Punzo R, Strino A, Acone R, Affuso G, Read J (2017b). General practitioners' beliefs about people with schizophrenia and whether they should be subject to discriminatory treatment when in medical hospital: the mediating role of dangerousness perception. *American Journal of Orthopsychiatry 87*: 559–566.

Magliano L, Read J, Rinaldi A et al (2016). The influence of causal explanations and diagnostic labeling on psychology students' beliefs about treatments, prognosis, dangerousness and unpredictability in schizophrenia. *Community Mental Health Journal 52*: 361–369.

Magliano L, Strino A, Punzo R, Acone R, Affuso G, Read J (2017a). Effects of the diagnostic label 'schizophrenia', actively used or passively accepted, on general practitioners' views of this disorder. *International Journal of Social Psychiatry 63*: 224–234.

Martinez A, Piff P, Mendoza-Denton R, Hinshaw S (2011). The power of a label: ascribed humanity and social rejection. *Journal of Social and Clinical Psychology 30*: 1–23.

May J (1922). *Mental Diseases*. Boston: Gorham.

Morrison A (2013). Cognitive therapy for people experiencing psychosis. In: Read J, Dillon J (eds). *Models of Madness* (2nd ed). London: Routledge (pp319–335).

Neil S, Pitt L, Kilbride M, Welford M, Northard S, Selwood W, Morrison A (2009). The questionnaire about the process of recovery (QPR): a measurement tool developed in collaboration with service users. *Psychosis: Psychological, Social and Integrative Approaches 1*: 145–155.

Penn D, Nowlin-Drummond A (2001). Politically correct labels and schizophrenia. *Schizophrenia Bulletin 27*: 197–203.

Pilgrim D (2000). Psychiatric diagnosis: more questions than answers. *Psychologist 13*: 302–305.

Pitt L, Kilbride M, Welford M (2007). Researching recovery from psychosis: a user-led project. *Psychiatric Bulletin 31*: 55–60.

Rattehalli R, Jayaram M, Smith M (2010). Risperidone versus placebo for schizophrenia. *Cochrane Database of Systematic Reviews* 20 January: CD006918.

Read J (2013a). The invention of 'schizophrenia: Kraepelin and Bleuler. In: Read J, Dillon J (eds). *Models of Madness* (2nd ed). London: Routledge (pp20–33).

Read J (2013b). Does 'schizophrenia' exist? Reliability and validity. In: Read J, Dillon J (eds). *Models of Madness* (2nd ed). London: Routledge (pp47–61).

Read J (2013c). Biological psychiatry's lost cause: The 'schizophrenic brain'. In: Read J, Dillon J (eds). *Models of Madness* (2nd ed). London: Routledge (pp62–71).

Read J (2013d) Childhood adversity and psychosis: from heresy to certainty. In: Read J, Dillon J (eds). *Models of Madness* (2nd ed). London: Routledge (pp249–275).

Read J (2010). Can poverty drive you mad? 'Schizophrenia', socio-economic status and the case for primary prevention. *New Zealand Journal of Psychology 39*: 7–19.

Read J (2008). Schizophrenia, drug companies and the internet. *Social Science and Medicine 66*: 99–109.

Read J, Dillon J (2013). Creating evidence-based, effective and humane mental health services: overcoming barriers to a paradigm shift. In: Read J, Dillon J (eds). *Models of Madness* (2nd ed). London: Routledge (pp392-407).

Read J, Fosse R, Moskowitz A, Perry B (2014). The traumagenic neurodevelopmental model of psychosis revisited. *Neuropsychiatry 4*: 65–79.

Read J, Harper D, Tucker I, Kennedy A (2018a). Do mental health services identify child abuse and neglect? A systematic review. *International Journal of Mental Health Nursing 27*: 7-19.

Read J, Harper D, Tucker I, Kennedy A (2018b). How do mental health services respond when child abuse or neglect become known? A literature review. *International Journal of Mental Health Nursing* 5 June. doi.org/10.1111/inm.12498

Read J, Haslam N, Magliano L (2013). Prejudice, stigma and 'schizophrenia': tThe role of bio-genetic ideology. In: Read J, Dillon J (eds). *Models of Madness* (2nd ed). London: Routledge (pp157–177).

Read J, Haslam N, Sayce L, Davies E (2006). Prejudice and schizophrenia: a review of the 'Mental illness is an Illness like any other' approach. *Acta Psychiatrica Scandinavica 114*: 303–318.

Read J, Johnstone L, Taitimu M (2013). Psychosis, poverty and ethnicity. In: Read J, Dillon J (eds). *Models of Madness* (2nd ed). London: Routledge (pp191–209).

Read J, Law A (1999). The relationship of causal beliefs and contact with users of mental health services to attitudes to the 'mentally ill'. *International Journal of Psychiatry 45*: 216–229.

Read J, Magliano L, Beavan V (2013). Public beliefs about the causes of 'schizophrenia': bad things happen and can drive you crazy. In: Read J, Dillon J (eds). *Models of Madness* (2nd ed). London: Routledge (pp143–156).

Read J, Sanders P (2010). *A Straight Talking Introduction to the Causes of Mental Health Problems.* Ross-on-Wye: PCCS Books.

Read J, Bentall RP, Johnstone L, Fosse R, Bracken P (2013). Electroconvulsive therapy. In: Read J, Dillon J (eds). *Models of Madness* (2nd ed). London: Routledge (pp90-104).

Riedel-Heller S, Matschinger H, Angermeyer M (2005). Mental disorders – who and what might help? Help-seeking and treatment preferences of the lay public. *Social Psychiatry and Psychiatric Epidemiology 40*: 167–174.

Roe A (1949). Integration of personality theory and clinical practice. *American Psychologist 44*: 806–815.

Rosenhan D (1975). On being sane in insane places. *Science 179*: 250–258.

Schomerus G, Evans-Lacko S, Rüsch N, Mojtabai R, Angermeyer M, Thornicroft G (2015). Collective levels of stigma and national suicide rates in 25 European countries. *Epidemiology and Psychiatric Sciences 24*: 166–171.

Schulze B, Richter-Werling M, Matschinger H, Angermeyer M (2003). Crazy? So what! Effects of a school project on students' attitudes towards people with schizophrenia. *Acta Psychiatrica Scandinavica 107*:142–150.

Slater L (2004). *Opening Skinner's Box.* New York: Norton.

Stevens L, Spencer H, Turkington D (2017). Identifying four subgroups of trauma in psychosis: vulnerability, psychopathology, and treatment. *Frontiers in Psychiatry 8*: 21.

Sweeney A, Clement S, Filson B, Kennedy A (2016). Trauma-informed mental healthcare in the UK: What is it and how can we further its development? *Mental Health Review Journal, 21*: 174–192.

Thomas P, Seebohm P, Wallcraft J, Kalathil J, Fernando S (2013). Personal consequences of the diagnosis of schizophrenia: a preliminary report from the inquiry into the schizophrenia label. *Mental Health and Social Inclusion 17*(3): 135–138.

Thornicroft G, Brohan E, Rose D, Sartorius N, Leese M, INDIGO Study Group (2009). Global pattern of experienced and anticipated discrimination against people with schizophrenia. *Lancet 373*: 408–415.

Torrey E (1987). Prevalence studies in schizophrenia. *British Journal of Psychiatry150*: 598–608.

Ucok A, Brohan E, Rose D et al (2012). Anticipated discrimination among people with schizophrenia. *Acta Psychiatrica Scandinavica 125*: 77–83.

van Os J, Verdoux H (2003). Diagnosis and classification of schizophrenia: categories versus dimensions, distributions versus disease. In: Murray R, Jones P, Susser E, van Os J, Cannon M (eds). *The Epidemiology of Schizophrenia*. Cambridge: Cambridge University Press (pp364–410).

Varese F, Smeets F, Drukker M et al (2012). Childhood adversities increase the risk of psychosis: a meta-analysis of patient-control, prospective- and cross-sectional cohort studies. *Schizophrenia Bulletin 38*: 661–671.

Weinmann S, Read J, Aderhold V (2009). The influence of antipsychotics on mortality in schizophrenia: a systematic review. *Schizophrenia Research 113*: 1–11.

Whitaker R (2010). *Anatomy of an Epidemic: magic bullets, psychiatric drugs, and the astonishing rise of mental illness in America*. New York, NY: Crown.

World Health Organization (2018). *International Classification of Diseases* (11th edn). Geneva: WHO.

World Health Organisation (1973). *The International Pilot Study of Schizophrenia, Vol 1*. Geneva: WHO.

Yamaguchi S, Mizuno M, Ojio Y, Sawada U, Matsunaga A, Ando S, Koike S (2017). Associations between renaming schizophrenia and stigma-related outcomes: a systematic review. *Psychiatry and Clinical Neurosciences 71*: 347–362.

Yanos P, Roe D, Lysaker P (2010). The impact of illness identity on recovery from severe mental illness. *American Journal of Psychiatric Rehabilitation 13*: 73–93.

Zigler E, Phillips L (1961). Psychiatric diagnosis: a critique. *Journal of Social and Abnormal Psychology 63*: 607–618.

9 | Resistance, rebellion, resilience and recovery

Akima Thomas

Women's subjection is carved deep into the rise of male-dominant rule, the matrilineal heritage abandoned and its immensity obliterated from the female psyche. The dominance of patriarchy was not a momentous, bloody, watershed event but rather a discreet, slow, insidious dripping of ideology, propagated throughout society.

This chapter will explore the history of the pathologisation of women and how that has been translated into shaming and blaming women and girl survivors of violence as the cause of their own distress (Caplan, 2005). It will end with a description of the Women and Girls Network and its work to restore women's sense of pride, strength and agency and empower them as survivors, not victims, of state-sanctioned male violence.

Women as 'mad' and 'bad'

The pathologisation of womanhood has a long tradition. It is entwined with the development of psychiatry and is tasked with the containment and elimination of society's undesirables. 'Hysteria' was the malady of preference bestowed on women during the 18th and 19th centuries. The history of 'hysteria' can be traced back to the ancient Egyptians and Greeks. It was used by Plato and Hippocrates to describe a range of female disorders believed to be linked to the spontaneous wandering of the uterus around the body (Ussher, 2013). However, the term really came into prominence with the alienists and the advent of the psychology and psychiatry professions, led by the likes of Briquet, Charcot, Janet and Freud. They made the link with 'hysteria' as a symbolic representation of trauma. Freud initiated the boldest leap when he identified 'hysterical symptoms' as testimony of sexual violence. He later recanted this causal link, giving way to social pressures and the maintenance of patriarchal status quo, and it was buried for another 100 years (Herman, 1992; Shaw & Proctor, 2005; Ussher, 2013).

The framing of women as 'mad' and/or 'bad' has always been led by the medical fraternity through its creation of diagnostic characteristics that reflect and reinforce the patriarchal social order (Higginbotham, 2017). Feminists argue that diagnoses are artificially and socially constructed systems developed to obscure and misrepresent the reality of women's lives. The psychiatric over-emphasis on objective scientific reasoning is misleading; rather, the biomedical model is inherently biased and intent on maintaining the status quo and reinforcing the acceptable socially permissible version of womanhood (Shaw & Proctor, 2005).

An illustration of the might of the psychiatric institution and its insistence on women's conformity is evident in the diagnostic category of 'personality disorder', and in particular 'borderline personality disorder' (BPD). As 'hysteria' fell out of vogue during the 20th century, it was seamlessly replaced by 'BPD', a term originally coined by Adolf Stern in 1938 to describe people with 'mild schizophrenia' and considered 'on the border' between 'neurosis' and 'psychosis' (Shaw & Proctor, 2005).

'BPD' is a highly feminised diagnosis – more than 75% of those diagnosed are women (Ussher, 2013). A catch-all diagnosis, it continues to be controversial, with considerable criticism led by feminists (Becker, 1997). For many, the diagnosis represents biased value judgements about women, built on a powerful social construction of 'normality' and 'abnormality', 'sanity' and 'madness', usually adjudicated by an individual psychiatrist (Brown, 2018). The diagnosis is heavily biased in favour of male definitions of 'normality' and encapsulates society's contemporary delineations of what is considered permissible behaviour in women. The 'BPD' criteria define the boundaries of tolerated behaviour; when the designated lines are crossed, as in women displaying anger or other intense emotion, their conduct is pathologised as 'mad', 'disordered', inappropriate. Normalcy is a tightly scripted role, defined from a male perspective, setting out what are deemed healthy behaviours and relationships for a woman. There is no consideration of gender differences in socialisation processes or reference to the influence of societal expectations governing the strict gender-coding of roles. Efforts to survive, such as eating disorders and self-injury, under the gaze of 'BPD', are encrypted as 'deviant' and 'pathological', and punished.

Similarly, 'premenstrual dysphoric disorder' pathologises the very essence of wombhood (Ussher, 2013). As with 'BPD', the unacceptability of anger is a key determinant for this diagnosis and reinforces society's perception that anger is outside of the permissible range of emotional responses for women. The misogynistic influence creates an unfortunate caricature of women and her raging hormones as unpredictable, unreliable and dangerous – a viewpoint that fits conveniently with social norms intended to restrict women's access to power and equality of opportunities (Ussher, 2013).

The myth of the tranquil woman

Psychiatry has always led the misogynistic framing of women as weak, vulnerable, 'neurotic' and insidiously 'mad' and 'bad'. The biomedical world has consistently regarded womanhood as a departure from the male norm that requires treatment with pharmaceuticals. During the 19th and 20th centuries, drugs such as morphine, opium, cocaine, cannabis, laughing gas and barbiturates were freely prescribed to treat a host of so-called female complaints, from gynaecological symptoms to 'nerves' and 'anxiety'. Pharmaceuticals were also dispensed covertly for other reasons. Following the Second World War, the state insisted women left the workforce and returned to the home to resume domestic duties, to free up jobs for the returning soldiers. The medics and psychiatrists supported this retreat by the wholesale sedation of women with prescriptions for Valium and other barbiturates, coyly described as 'mothers' little helpers' because of their alleged ability to assuage the pressures of motherhood, home-making and other 'female' problems (Brown, 2018).

The challenge to this wholesale sedation of women was led in the 1960s by feminists like Betty Friedan, who challenged the pharmaceutical industry's generalisation of the 'problem that has no name' – her label for the fatigue and feelings of emptiness that afflicted many housewives treated with tranquillisers. Friedan asserted that women's predisposition to 'nervous illness' had less to do with 'anxiety' and 'depression' and more to do with repressed frustration with their unfulfilled lives (Worell & Remer, 2003). The women's liberation movement during the 1960s and 1970s demanded equality and asserted women's rights to full and equal participation in society. It brought male violence against women out of the closet of the domestic and private domain and into the public's consciousness through the political act of breaking the silence. The medical response was swift, numbing and silencing, as evidenced by the startling statistic that, from 1969–1982, Valium was the most prescribed drug in the northern hemisphere (Brown, 2018).

Violence against women and girls

A feminist analysis views patriarchal dominance as maintained through consistent re-enactments of power. Sexual terrorism and other forms of interpersonal violence are its most pertinent forms for modelling power-over and strengthening male supremacy. All women are targeted through a web of fear, with palpable daily reminders of dominance intended to reinforce male privilege and restrict women's agency and freedom.

Essential to maintaining the system are the creation and propagation of misinformation and distorted meaning, which function to preserve the façade.

The medical model, and psychiatry in particular, have been useful allies in the concealment of reality, from Freud and his portrayal of women as fantasists to targeted diagnosis depicting women as unreliable, flawed, with unstable personalities, to be treated with drugs and locked up in asylums. As with any system of dominance, the victim has to be held to blame. Hence, under patriarchy, survivors of male violence and abuse have been regarded as the cause of the perpetrators' offending behaviour. The blame-game places emphasis on the survivor's personal characteristics, her behaviour, location, dress choice and consumption of drugs and/or alcohol. Her consent is presumed because she didn't fight or run, or she stayed in/returned to the abusive relationship. The perpetrator is pushed to the background, obscured by society's efficient sanitising processes (Herman, 1992).

Hiding the reality and seeking truth

Feminists argue that patriarchy's propaganda has been effectively distilled into women's psyche from birth. A thread of self-doubt, acceptance of blame and sense of responsibility for the other and their actions is tightly woven into and intrinsically forms part of women's identity (Brown, 2018; Worell & Remer 2003). The disconnection with the reality of gender-based violence relies on this to ensure women feel accountable for the violence inflicted on them, trapping them in a vicious cycle of blame and shame by sanctioning their sole responsibility for their distress.

The diagnostic frameworks and the de-contextualisation of the harm women endure ensure the injuries of gender-based violence are individualised and coded as women's 'madness' because of their 'badness'. We become the scapegoat for society's evils (Herman, 1992; Ussher, 2013). But what women have is incurable; the only treatments on offer are chemical silencers, so even if she does scream, who will hear? Certainly the diagnosis of 'BPD' has become the dustbin diagnosis of mental health services, with its pernicious labelling of women as manipulative, attention-seeking, aggressive, clinging – a toxic contagion to be avoided at all costs by clinicians (Brown, 2018; Higginbotham, 2017).

Trauma

Trauma has entered the psychotherapy/psychology lexicon as a key cause of much emotional distress. It is unquestionably a valuable way to contextualise human suffering, especially in relation to violence against women and girls. However, we need to be wary here and question whether the construct conceals more than it reveals. The use of trauma narratives is appealing but there is an obvious convergence with other medical constructs – the same individualising of the problem and ignoring of the role of the perpetrator as the source of harm.

It can be argued that trauma models over-emphasise the importance of neurological factors and present a distorted reality of what needs to be fixed. Negated within the trauma models is any attention to the woman's external reality and an understanding that the brain occupies a body that is racialised, genderised, classified and exposed to myriad oppressions (Reynolds, 2014). Violence and oppression are in the real world, not within survivors' brains, and we must not allow this to be forgotten. Language is a powerful communicator and must be scrutinised to ensure it does not reinforce societal agendas that deny, minimise or rationalise violence against women and girls and its effects. Understanding the effects of violence must recognise and affirm the harm and distress to survivors and locate responsibility firmly with the perpetrator. Attempts to help survivors must be nested in an awareness of the threats posed by the real world that the survivor inhabits.

Women and Girls Network

Women and Girls Network (WGN) was born from the womb of feminist activism, founded to challenge the social constructs that seek to silence, blame, deny, minimise, justify and obscure women's experiences of gendered violence. WGN was created through feminist activism; social justice is reflected and integrated into every aspect of our work, providing a holistic perspective that validates and exposes the broader social context of the lives of survivors of violence. Our aim is to deconstruct the political and social environment and position WGN as an alternative to essentially misogynistic man-stream theories and traditional biomedical models of working with violence against women and girls.

Embodying feminist practice is a bold statement and the process begins with us, the practitioners, and our authenticity in the work. This requires consideration and analysis of power dynamics, staying consistently attuned to power imbalances and finding meaningful solutions to dismantle hierarchies and preserve survivors' autonomy to create vibrant collaborative spaces of solidarity. Our work is not based on objectivity and clinical distancing, but on self-involvement through open, transparent and honest dialogue in which we are standing in solidarity alongside survivors. Collective identification through appropriate sharing of experiences of oppression and discrimination is essential to the mutuality that lies at the heart of our dialogues, creating spaces for healing and transformation.

Gender responsive approach

It is essential to our way of working to ensure we use a wide lens to capture the totality of survivors' experience, including their past and present socio-economic and political external environment that influences and shapes their internal worlds. These two elements are intrinsically linked and influence the direction of care and the potential for change – in feminist terms, the personal is political. Working with violence against women and girls demands that we are not neutral, that we adopt an ethical, political and moral stance. We refuse to maintain the status quo by supporting functional women to function in dysfunctional spaces. We seek to change the real conditions of women's lives, not to help them to adapt to oppression. We support them to stand out, not fit in (Brown, 2018; Reynolds, 2014).

Our work seeks transformation and social justice because we understand the reality and toxicity endemic within patriarchy. We see through the veil of disguises offered by state systems. We detach violence against women and girls from the culture of individualised blame and hold the state accountable. Contextualising violence against women and girls within an ecological frame holds the individual perpetrator responsible but also holds to account the powerful social influences of community, state and the system of patriarchy, with its legislation, policy and criminal justice system and the weak sanctions that serve to condone and legitimise men's violence.

This clarity about the causes of survivors' distress is vital to our work. We reject diagnostic frameworks such as 'BPD' that function to pathologise women and obscure the reality of the violence inflicted on us (Ussher, 2013). As feminists, we critique patriarchal rule as a highly toxic environment where women struggle to thrive. The daily micro-aggressions experienced by women contribute to a lifetime of macro-aggression that limits opportunities and drives gender inequality. The more women accumulate 'isms', the further marginalised we become, which in turn influences the responses we can expect from the criminal justice and healthcare systems, the diagnostic labels we are given and interventions we are offered. Intersectionality is a way to make sense of these myriad forms of oppression.

Resistance and freedom fighters

Resistance under patriarchy is usually understood as physically fighting back. Women and girl survivors of violence do not fit this male construct of resistance. However, women always resist; as Reynolds says (2014), they do so spontaneously, in the moment, with strategies based on intelligence and wisdom, to secure their survival.

WGN works from a strengths-based approach. Our aim is to enable women's rediscovery, reimagining and reconnection with their true, authentic selves in order to nurture a detachment and liberation from the perpetrator's aggression and intrusion into their core self. This requires more than a focus on the witnessing of traumatic events and tracking of trauma symptoms. As feminist activists, our work invites a dialogical model of communication and exploration of the multiple strands and interpretation of the trauma events, with particular emphasis on identifying sites of resistance (Brown, 2018; Reynolds,

2014). We are mindful not to be dogmatic in our interpretation of a survivor's narrative. However, our work aims to challenge the usual social constructs of the survivor as passive victim by validating and affirming what she has done to resist and survive.

This attention to discovering and celebrating survivors' strategies of resistance is at the heart of our work and the changes it achieves are obvious, with survivors noticeably coming back into their bodies. We see physical responses, such as a straightening of the spine, inhalation of breath inflating the chest, and facial muscles relaxing as they recount how incredible it is that they have survived and that they continue to survive. This physical manifestation of pride and dignity is partnered with an inner process of transformation, igniting the survivor's narrative to include actions she can take. There is a shift from the acknowledgment that 'I am alive and 'This is what I did to survive' to 'This is what I can now do'. This is a powerful antidote to the constriction inherent in the biomedical model. This more expansive view places the survivor centrally within the story of her life and amplifies her powers of proactive resistance, her capability to restore and reclaim, her autonomy and agency. This is crucial for the survivor's transformation and healing. We practitioners and social activists then become witnesses and allies to this potential, rather than merely the audience, passively witnessing suffering.

Holistic empowerment recovery model

We have evolved the Holistic Empowerment Recovery (HER) model as a framework to meet survivors' need for a wraparound service that provides them with an inclusive therapeutic journey that can respond to the breadth of their needs.

The model is guided by an ethos of personal empowerment that aims to restore survivors' sense of agency, power and control. The work is structured to extend and enhance survivor's capabilities and frames their strategies for survival and adaptation to the trauma response within a strengths-based model. Central to the model is an inclusive response designed to meet the needs and aspirations of survivors from traditionally marginalised and excluded communities, to ensure a sensitive and appropriate response.

The model comprises seven domains that operate at differing levels of intensity and in no set sequence, so they are responsive to the needs of the survivor (see figure 1).

Rebel nation

There are no public memorials erected as testimonies to the atrocities of violence against women and girls and countless lives lost. However, survivors work throughout the sector delivering services and supporting other survivors. By

Figure 1: Holistic empowerment recovery model

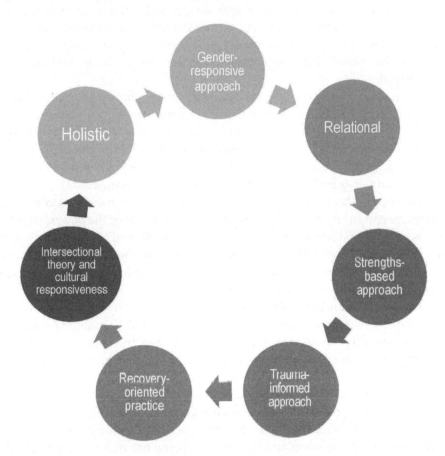

this beautiful transcendence of and through their experiences, survivors become the living monuments and testimonies to their own resistance and ambitions for recovery. At WGN, we are increasingly moving away from the professionalisation of the trauma industry and are intent on emancipation structures, appreciating survivors as liberators and advocates. This has meant stepping back from our professional status and supporting survivors to co-produce projects as experts by experience. At WGN, survivors lead on developing and facilitating group spaces and co-delivering training. WGN is also partnered with Million Women Rise, a feminist social activist movement intent on the eradication of male violence through peace, solidarity and revolutionary love.

Badra's story

Badra was a 32-year-old survivor of childhood sexual violence and adult rape who came to us with a long history of mental health service use and 15 years of diagnoses, including 'ADHD', 'emotionally unstable BPD', 'eating disorder' and 'substance misuse'. She was at first disappointed and frustrated that we didn't give her yet another diagnosis during the initial assessment. She had so internalised these diagnostic frameworks that they had become how she defined and described herself. Her symptoms had come to obscure Badra and her place in the world.

From these unsteady beginnings, our relationship with Badra began tentatively to grow, although our dance of synchronicity was often clumsy, leaving me at times feeling as if I were hippy-dippy and totally out of touch with real life. However, Badra gradually began to unfold, revealing a deeply rooted self-hatred. She saw herself as inherently evil and 'bad', and believed this was why so many bad things had happened to her; it was her punishment.

Our central task was to listen, hold and tentatively invite her to recount alternative narratives. We used psychoeducation to challenge the powerful myths and scripts around sexual violence that place blame and responsibility with survivors. Badra responded well to these discussions about responsibility and consent where we unmasked the reality of sexual violence, and this eventually interrupted her blame-and-shame cycle.

However, this understanding still left the agonising 'Why didn't I?' questions: 'Why didn't I stop it/tell someone/run/hit him?' She saw her failure to resist as synonymous with compliance and consent. Our response was to reframe and re-interpret her inactivity as active resistance, using questions such as: 'What strategies did you use to survive?' These opened up a whole new dialogue that revealed Badra's resistance strategies that had ensured she stayed safe and alive – her strategies to prevent assaults in childhood, such as minimising times when she was alone with the perpetrator, disconnecting and psychically hiding herself during assaults, being silent and still but occupying her mind by escaping into revenge fantasises, minimising violence by saying the perpetrator's name and using humour to keep him calm. The list was phenomenal and showed that Badra had never been a willing, compliant or passive 'victim' but had developed an elaborate range of proactive strategies to minimise the impact of violence and keep safe.

This naming/identifying and telling of her resistance strategies was immensely cathartic for Badra, and her physical presence changed with these new realisations. She was able to connect with a sense of pride and became aware of her strengths, abilities and resilience. As she became more connected to her true and authentic self, the psychiatric labels had less relevance and she became increasingly resentful of the way she had been silenced and forced to withdraw from the world and seen as the cause of her own problems.

As she healed, her world expanded, and she was able to be more present in it. With her new-found sense of confidence and freedom, she joined Million Women Rise and found a collective purpose, strength, encouragement and support to live her life differently. However, it would be wrong to present this as an idealised picture of recovery. It is a very brief snapshot of a complex therapeutic journey that took more than a year. Badra continues to be challenged and distressed by her experiences; she still faces challenges and struggles to live life as she would choose. The effects of a lifetime of abuse and psychiatric mistreatment do not heal so easily.

The crimes of gender-based violence are atrocities against humanity. However, survivors have always been rebels, transforming their pain into becoming agents of change, driving the feminist movement to create theory and practice that challenges patriarchal neoliberalism's insistence on maintaining the status quo of social inequality. Million Women Rise, Me Too and Time's Up are all examples of campaigns led by survivors who refuse to be silenced and demand justice. These are the rebels with a cause.

References

Becker D (1997). *Through the Looking Glass: women and borderline personality disorder.* New York, NY: Perseus Books.

Brown L (2018). *Feminist Therapy.* Washington DC: American Psychological Association.

Caplan PJ (2005). *The Myth of Women's Masochism.* iUniverse.

Herman JL (1992). *Trauma and Recovery: the aftermath of violence – from domestic abuse to political terror.* New York, NY: Basic Books.

Higginbotham J (2017). *Borderline Personality Disorder: patriarchal boundaries of sanity, self and sex.* [Online.] Academia. www.academia.edu/2080856/Borderline_Personality_Disorder_Patriarchal_Boundaries_of_Sanity_Self_and_Sex (accessed 25 June 2019).

Reynolds V (2014). Centering ethics in group supervision: fostering cultures of critique and structuring safety. *The International Journal of Narrative Therapy and Community Work 1*: 1–13.

Shaw C, Proctor G (2005). Women at the margins: a critique of the diagnosis of borderline personality disorder. *Feminism and Psychology 15*(4): 483–490.

Ussher J (2013). Diagnosing difficult women and pathologising femininity: gender bias in psychiatric nosology. *Feminism and Psychology 23*(1): 63–69.

Worell J, Remer P (2003). *Feminist Perspectives in Therapy: empowering diverse women* (2nd ed). Hoboken, NJ: John Wiley & Sons.

10 | Why words can harm your mental health

Gary Sidley

The popular 'sticks and stones' children's rhyme insists that words 'can never harm you' and that we should take little notice of them. Urging us all to focus on actions rather than words seems like sound advice. We tend to be more impressed by a person who 'walks the walk' rather than one who 'talks the talk'. And, given the fundamental flaws in the ways that Western societies respond to human suffering – for example, the widespread human-rights violations and gross overuse of psychiatric drugs – it may, at first, seem hugely pedantic to be highlighting the importance of language. Nonetheless, in this chapter I will argue that words are an important element in our mission to improve the wellbeing of those whose lives are blighted by emotional distress and overwhelm.

After illustrating how a focus on language can evoke criticism from some mental health professionals and service users, I will describe the power of words to impact on two crucial components of a sufferer's experience: stigma and so-called therapeutic optimism about the prospect of change. In addition – and perhaps of greater importance – I will discuss the way that language can significantly influence the viability of innovative alternatives to the dominant biomedical approach. Specific examples will be offered to illustrate the assumptions underlying terms and phrases commonly heard within the world of psychiatry and mental health. My central argument is that the unthinking use of biomedical language perpetuates the status quo, maintaining the dominance of biological psychiatry. Thus, it is important that we all remain aware of the implicit messages associated with the language we use as they may not always be congruent with our intended aims.

Indignation towards the 'thought police'

People can often react angrily towards those who they believe are trying to influence their speech. A stark example of this concerns the reactions to a document published in 2015 by the Division of Clinical Psychology (DCP) within the British Psychological Society (the professional association for practising psychologists in the UK), titled *Guidelines on Language in Relation to Functional Psychiatric Diagnosis*. Despite the stated purpose of these guidelines being restricted to encouraging clinical psychologists to consider using non-medical language when writing about human distress, the scale of indignant protest from some quarters implied that we were witnessing the imposition of thought censorship of Orwellian proportion.

The reactions to these language guidelines, as vented via blogs, Twitter and other forms of social media, encompassed a range of grievances: discouraging diversity in language use; attempting to police the mind; discounting an individual's preferred form of expression. Others felt patronised by the document's recommendations or suspected the psychology profession was trying to impose its self-promoting view of the world.

It is not only those sympathetic to biomedical psychiatry who reject the assertion that words are important when describing human suffering. For example, I am a moderator on the 'Drop the Disorder!' Facebook group[1] – a collective of service users, professionals and others committed to promoting a radical alternative to the dominant 'illness like any other' approach to emotional pain and overwhelm. In this role, I have witnessed disparaging reactions to posts highlighting the importance of language. One accusation has been that discussions about the words we use is an 'intellectual' debate, an academic argument mainly involving professionals locked in a university ivory tower, immune from the harsh realities of the real world. While many people are suffering systematic abuse, they argue, this pedantic conversation about language is just an academic exercise that changes nothing for the victims of the current psychiatric system who are crying out for action and support. The overarching message from these dissenters is something like, 'I don't care what you call me, or my distress – words change nothing.'

Those opposed to devoting time to exploring the impact of language may fail to see the link between words and the way people in distress are treated by services and society as a whole. Such an oversight is, in some instances, perfectly understandable; if you, or a loved one, are currently suffering incarceration and enforced drugging within a psychiatric unit, a focus on language use would be low on the list of priorities. Yet I continue to believe that the association between words and service responses is significant and insidious.

---

1. www.adisorder4everyone.com/new-facebook-group

Why do words matter?

There is now widespread acceptance that some words traditionally used to describe people in receipt of psychiatric services are derogatory and unacceptable. At their most blatant, references to such terms as 'psycho', 'schizo' and 'loony' are rightfully recognised as misleading and offensive. A headline seen in *The Sun* newspaper in 2003, referring to boxer Frank Bruno's compulsory admission to psychiatric hospital as 'BONKERS BRUNO LOCKED UP', would now attract condemnation from all but the most bigoted (Nunn, 2014). However, the more subtle consequences of what might appear to be benign language are arguably more damaging to people struggling with emotional distress and overwhelm, particularly in the long term.

One important example is the link between biomedical language and stigma – 'a sign of disgrace or discredit which sets a person apart from others' (Byrne, 2000: 65). People tagged as displaying psychiatric problems often subsequently endure prejudice and discrimination. The negative consequences of this bigotry include inflated perceptions of their dangerousness and unpredictability, exclusion from valued roles, more social isolation, and targeting for harassment and abuse (see Sidley, 2015: 39–43, for a review). In recognition of this societal problem, a number of high-profile 'anti-stigma' campaigns have been implemented across the developed world. Regrettably, the 'illness like any other' explanations for human distress promoted in these public education initiatives will have exacerbated the levels of stigma within our society, with language making a significant contribution to this unintended consequence.

There is compelling evidence to suggest that explanations of human distress that give prominence to the role of genetic and biological 'abnormalities' tend to strengthen stigmatising attitudes while, in contrast, psychosocial explanations that highlight the role of adverse life experiences are likely to reduce them (Read et al, 2006; Longden & Read, 2017). In particular, holding biogenetic views about the cause of mental health problems will fuel a number of negative consequences for the sufferer, including a reluctance of others to form friendships with them (Golding et al, 1975; Read & Harre, 2001); inflated perceptions of dangerousness and unpredictability (Read & Harre, 2001; Walker & Read, 2002), and a greater risk of being treated more harshly (Mehta & Farina, 1997). The words we use to describe human suffering and overwhelm will significantly shape the recipient's explanatory model and, in so doing, either strengthen or dilute stigmatising beliefs. Thus, use of diagnostic labels (such as 'schizophrenia' or 'bipolar disorder') and medical terminology ('symptoms', 'treatments', 'diagnosis') will propagate biogenetic understandings and, by doing so, encourage prejudice and discrimination towards psychiatric service users.

In addition to influencing the levels of discrimination endured by people suffering emotional distress, there is evidence to suggest that our vocabulary might impact on the degree of optimism about the prospect of recovery. At the point of contact with psychiatric services, a person is typically overwhelmed and finding it difficult to imagine a positive future. As such, maintaining hope is an essential aim of any effective response. Unhelpfully, the language of psychiatric diagnosis can heighten perceptions of the seriousness of a person's problems (Cormack & Furnham, 1998), lead to an underestimation of their social skills (Read & Haslam, 2004), and fuel pessimism with regards to a successful outcome (Angermeyer & Matschinger, 1996). Thus, resorting to psychiatric labels may dampen expectations of a positive resolution.

The link between language and innovation

Those of us who are critical of the biological psychiatry's 'illness like any other' approach to human suffering often ask ourselves two intriguing questions. First, given the robust evidence base suggesting that traditional psychiatry's biomedical interventions are only modestly effective and often damaging, why do they continue to dominate? Second, why do attempts to introduce innovative alternatives to the options offered by traditional psychiatry often end in failure, with the 'new' idea ultimately diluted, corrupted or ignored altogether? (This frustration will be recognised by anyone who has striven to establish psychosocial practices within core psychiatric services.) Although there are likely to be a number of explanations for why innovation is so difficult – for example, the vested interests of the psychiatry profession and the pharmaceutical industry, political convenience – language may be an important reason for the stubborn persistence of medicalised understandings of human suffering.

Boyle (2013) describes two main tactics used by traditional psychiatry to nullify alternative, non-biological approaches. The crudest strategy is 'invalidation', where the defender of the status quo resorts to ridicule and personal attacks. Examples of this form of attack – often deployed in blogs, media reports and opinion pieces – would include accusations that the innovators are 'self-promoters' or 'scientologists' or simply engaged in 'a turf war'. A recent, high-profile example of invalidation was when Jeffrey Lieberman (a former president of the American Psychiatric Association), in a radio interview, dismissed Bob Whitaker (a journalist and vocal critic of biological psychiatry) as a 'menace to society'. In this instance, Whitaker's crime was to make the evidence-based assertion that, in the long term, people suffering psychotic experiences did better without psychiatric drugs (Wipond, 2015). Although unpleasant, these attempts to invalidate the innovator are easy to repel and usually inflict no enduring damage on the credibility of the alternative proposal.

The second ploy to impede innovation – and the one where language may play a pivotal role – Boyle refers to as 'assimilation' (Boyle, 2013). The assimilation process involves the removal of the most radical aspects of the new idea so that what remains appears different from the dominant orthodoxy only in degree of emphasis. In the aftermath of this neutering, those seeking to protect the biomedical status quo can claim that the proposed innovation is not really 'new' and that the existing service is 'doing this already'.

Boyle persuasively argues that the words we use to describe our alternative approaches may determine their degree of immunity to assimilation. Adopting the language of physical illness when discussing innovative interventions to reduce emotional distress will render them more vulnerable to dilution. Thus, the habitual use of terms such as 'treatment', 'symptoms', 'relapse', 'disorders' and 'diagnosis' – typical of all professional groups currently working in psychiatric services – will convey the impression that any disagreement with biological psychiatry is only superficial: 'You provide psychological treatments of mental disorders, I'll provide drug treatments for mental disorders' (Boyle, 2013: 14).

Using language to promote alternatives to the biomedical paradigm

Before I go on to further explore the type of words that might aid the realisation of a paradigm shift in the way we respond to human distress, it is imperative that I emphasise a key point: I unequivocally respect the rights of people to use any words they think fit to describe their own suffering. Each individual who is struggling with emotional pain and overwhelm is uniquely positioned to try to make sense of their difficulties and convey them to others in language that best captures the experience. For example, if a person believes labelling the experience as an 'illness' seems to best capture its nature, so be it. Conversely, I believe that those wielding power as opinion shapers – professional bodies, mental health professionals, journalists, celebrities – carry a burden of responsibility not to mislead the general public about the nature of human suffering. It is with regard to this latter group that choice of language is important.

Language is organic, constantly changing. When I revisit articles or blogs that I wrote a few years ago, I often cringe at my choice of words. Furthermore, while there are unambiguous examples of biomedical terms oozing stigma and pessimism – 'chronic schizophrenia', for example – language choice can sometimes be a matter of personal preference. I deliver a workshop exploring the importance of language in relation to human suffering and one of the exercises involves asking the participants to opt for what they believe to be the most appropriate term for someone in contact with psychiatric services. Even though all the attendees, to varying degrees, display critical attitudes towards traditional psychiatric practice, there is always substantial disagreement as to the preferred descriptor. Some favour the term 'service user', while others – particularly those providing counselling and talking therapies – tend to prefer 'client'. Yet others suggest alternatives such as 'service receiver' or 'service participant'.

Nonetheless, it is important to recognise that our choice of words conveys implicit messages about the nature of human distress. Referring to misery as a consequence of 'brain disease', 'an illness like any other', 'biochemical imbalance', 'serotonin deficiency', 'a broken brain' or 'misfiring neurones' will inevitably propagate the myth that emotional pain is primarily the consequence of a brain disorder. Similarly, habitual use of diagnostic labels (such as 'bipolar disorder', 'depression', 'schizophrenia') and terminology extrapolated from the physical health world ('symptoms', 'treatments', 'diagnosis', 'relapse', 'illness') are all likely to further consolidate psychiatry's biomedical stranglehold on the way the Western world makes sense of and responds to emotional suffering. Thus, I believe it is imperative that those of us keen to promote an alternative paradigm, one that gives credence to the central role of life adversity in the emergence of human distress, should abandon the language of diagnosis and disorder.

As already discussed, the rejection of medical language in relation to emotional pain and overwhelm should help to counter stigma, promote optimism and render innovation within the psychiatric world more resistant to assimilation. But what form might this alternative language take?

How can we describe human suffering without recourse to biomedical language?

Medical discourse is so deeply embedded within Western culture that the use of its terminology often occurs automatically, without awareness or conscious effort – it is our common default position. Yet this resort to the language of physical illness colludes with, and perpetuates, the dominance of biological psychiatry in addressing human distress and overwhelm across the Western world. The generation of alternatives frequently requires prior reflection, and the non-medical descriptor may sometimes sound long and convoluted. Nonetheless, in light of the advantages of avoiding medical language, there are grounds to argue that it is worth the effort.

As proposed by the DCP's *Guidelines on Language in Relation to Functional Diagnoses* (BPS Division of Clinical Psychology, 2015), more benign alternatives can be generated to substitute for diagnostic labels and other biomedical terms. Instead of referring to 'mental illness' or 'mental disorder', the more neutral 'emotional distress' or 'emotional overwhelm' might be helpfully considered. Rather than 'patient' – a term that implies a passive recipient of medical expertise – we might substitute the term 'service user'. In place of 'symptom', 'treatment' and 'relapse', we might opt for 'difficulty', 'support' and 'return of emotional distress', respectively.

Given the arbitrary nature of many of the more common psychiatric diagnoses, nothing important is lost by avoiding such labels and, instead, describing the most prominent features of the presenting distress in everyday language. Thus, 'bipolar disorder' could become 'severe mood swings', and 'schizophrenia' could be exchanged for terms such as 'unusual beliefs' and/or 'hearing voices'. Similarly, neutral lay-person's language, offering a descriptive account of a service user's difficulties, would be preferable to the use of biomedical phrases in interprofessional communication. For example, instead of writing in someone's notes, 'Carol is displaying psychotic symptoms', you could record, 'Carol hears voices condemning her as dirty and worthless in the context of having been sexually abused as a child and adult'. The longer, descriptive communication avoids the disadvantages of biomedical language and makes the 'symptoms' intelligible by providing the backdrop of the person's life experiences – another important element in the struggle to shift the biomedical stranglehold (Boyle, 2013).

If we are to ensure our communications are perceived as relevant to the target audience, in some instances it may not be possible to avoid reference to a diagnostic label or other biomedical terms. In these circumstances, it may be helpful to acknowledge that these medicalised expressions represent one way of thinking about emotional distress rather than constituting an actual description of the phenomenon. This can be achieved by either using quote marks around the diagnostic label or preceding the biomedical term with a statement to indicate it represents just one way of making sense of the human experience under scrutiny – for example, 'What some professionals might consider to be "symptoms" of "depression"'. Adoption of this approach could help to counter the unhelpful tendency for the ubiquitous 'illness like any other' account of human suffering to be understood as a scientifically-confirmed reality.

Barriers to dropping the language of disorder

Indignant protest against the very idea that we should reflect on the language we use (discussed above) is not the only obstruction to change in the way we communicate about emotional distress. Arguably the most prominent barrier is the self-serving misinformation generated by those powerful stakeholders who benefit most from our biomedically dominated system: the pharmaceutical industry and the psychiatry profession.

The unholy alliance between drug companies and psychiatrists has been well documented (see Sidley, 2015: 146–165 for an overview). A language-assisted shift away from viewing human distress as a primary consequence of biological abnormalities (biochemical imbalances, brain defects and the like) would deliver a sizable dent to the profits of the drug industry. The rationale that drugs such as antidepressants and antipsychotics restore equilibrium to a diseased brain is a lucrative selling point for the drug industry, and widespread adoption of biomedical language aids this ongoing misrepresentation. One stark example concerns the antidepressant Paxil. When approved by the regulatory authorities as a treatment for severe shyness, the drug company's posters included the prompt, 'Imagine being allergic to people' (Moynihan, Heath & Henry, 2002).

The other institution to benefit from the 'illness like any other' approach to human suffering is the psychiatric profession. Abandoning the use of the language of physical health when describing distress would trigger questions about the legitimacy of psychiatrists occupying the top table of medicine, alongside the likes of oncology and cardiology specialists. Medicalised discourse helps protect the psychiatric profession from challenges to its expert status – so it's not surprising that they are so resistant to a shift towards alternative terminology.

Biomedical language is so deeply engrained in Western culture that the layperson may view it as benign, a description of how things are in actuality. Mental health charities and the mainstream media typically adopt biomedical language in their efforts to educate the public about the various kinds of emotional difficulties. Similarly, high-profile celebrities, in sharing their personal struggles with mental health problems, often use diagnostic labels as if these refer to identifiable brain diseases (for example, Stephen Fry's 'manic depression' or 'bipolar disorder'), or more generally indicate by their words that a brain abnormality is the primary cause (for example, Ruby Wax's utterances about a 'broken brain'). Given the ubiquitous use of these types of descriptions, the viewing public are unlikely to recognise the biomedical assumptions underlying them and will therefore fail to see any reason to question the appropriateness of the words used.

A further barrier to language change may derive from the privileges granted to people who have been given a psychiatric diagnosis. A label such as 'clinical depression' or 'schizophrenia' written on a health record can often be an essential requirement for accessing state benefits and a necessary passport for entry into specialist mental health services. In our medicalised society, references to 'illness' sound more serious and real in comparison with the alternatives that rely on descriptive, everyday language. Regrettably, within these long-established health and social care systems, the process for determining who is eligible for financial assistance and therapeutic support sometimes demands use of medical language. Therefore, until we witness a paradigm shift in the way the developed world makes sense of human suffering and overwhelm, a reliance on biomedical language will, to some extent, be necessary.

Final comments

Words matter. The language we use conveys information, often implicitly, about the way the world operates. With regard to human suffering and overwhelm, opinion shapers – mental health professionals, journalists, media celebrities – all have a responsibility not to mislead services users and the general public. Given the potential impact of language on stigma, hopefulness and the viability of innovative therapeutic interventions, it can be helpful for us all to reflect on the words we use and the underlying assumptions we are propagating. Attention to congruence is particularly important; it is untenable to claim to be promoting alternatives to the biomedical paradigm while espousing the language of diagnosis and disorder and thereby strengthening the hegemony of psychiatry.

To return to the 'sticks and stones' rhyme, our actions may – ultimately – be paramount, but our words can shape the beliefs and attitudes that determine how we behave.

References

Angermeyer M, Matschinger H (1996). The effects of labelling on the lay theory regarding schizophrenic disorders. *Social Psychiatry and Psychiatric Epidemiology 31*: 316–320.

Boyle M (2013). The persistence of medicalisation: is the presentation of alternatives part of the problem? In: Coles S, Keenan S, Diamond B (eds). *Madness Contested: power and practice*. Ross-on-Wye: PCCS Books (pp3–22).

British Psychological Society Division of Clinical Psychology (2015). *Guidelines on Language in Relation to Functional Diagnosis*. Leicester: British Psychological Society.

Byrne P (2000). Stigma of mental illness and ways of diminishing it. *Advances in Psychiatric Treatment 6*: 65–72.

Cormack S, Furnham A (1998). Psychiatric labelling, sex role stereotypes and beliefs about the mentally ill. *International Journal of Social Psychiatry 44*: 235–247.

Golding SL, Becker E, Sherman S, Rappaport J (1975). The Behavioural Expectations Scale: assessment of expectations for interaction with the mentally ill. *Journal of Consulting and Clinical Psychology 43*: 109.

Longden E, Read J (2017). 'People with problems, not patients with illnesses': using psychosocial frameworks to reduce the stigma of psychosis. *The Israel Journal of Psychiatry & Related Sciences 54*(1): 24–28.

Mehta S, Farina A (1997). Is being 'sick' really better? Effect of the disease view of mental disorder on stigma. *Journal of Social and Clinical Psychology 16*: 405–419.

Moynihan R, Heath I, Henry D (2002). Selling sickness: the pharmaceutical industry and disease mongering. *British Medical Journal 324*(7342): 886–991.

Nunn G (2014). Time to change the language we use about mental health. *The Guardian*; 28 February. [Online.] www.theguardian.com/media/mind-your-language/2014/feb/28/mind-your-language-mental-health (accessed 21 June 2019).

Read J, Harre N (2001). The role of biological and genetic causal beliefs in the stigmatisation of 'mental' patients. *Journal of Mental Health 10*: 223–235.

Read J, Haslam N (2004). Public opinion: bad things happen and can drive you crazy. In: Read J, Mosher LR, Bentall R (eds). *Models of Madness: psychological, social and biological approaches to schizophrenia*. London: Routledge (pp133–145).

Read J, Haslam N, Sayce L, Davies E (2006). Prejudice and schizophrenia: a review of the 'mental illness is an illness like any other' approach. *Acta Psychiatrica Scandinavica 114*(5): 303–318.

Sidley G (2015). *Tales from the Madhouse: an insider critique of psychiatric services*. Monmouth: PCCS Books.

Walker I, Read J (2002). The differential effectiveness of psycho-social and bio-genetic causal explanations in reducing negative attitudes towards 'mental illness'. *Psychiatry 65*: 313–325.

Wipond R (2015). *Lieberman Calls Whitaker 'A Menace to Society'*. [Online.] Mad in America; 26 April. www.madinamerica.com/2015/04/lieberman-calls-whitaker-menace-society/ (accessed 21 June 2019).

11 | Offensive pathways: the 'personality disorder' construct and the over-responsibilisation of incarcerated women

Robyn Timoclea

Receiving a diagnosis of 'borderline personality disorder' ('BPD') at the age of 17 was one of the worst things that happened to me. As a survivor of childhood multiple perpetrator rape, I expected support and compassion when I entered the mental health system; what I experienced was a bizarre and oppressive form of pseudo-medicalised victim blaming. While writing this chapter, I realised that I have spent more of my life in the UK mental health system than I have outside of it. The impact of this on my identity as a citizen (or, rather, not feeling like a citizen) cannot be underestimated or even fully articulated; it has shaped and continues to shape who I am as a woman and my perceived place in society. How much more so, then, for women who have experienced a 'BPD' diagnosis as well as incarceration in forensic institutions.

This chapter will begin with critical consideration of the diagnosis of 'BPD' before moving on to the situation for incarcerated women. I will draw on my lived experience of the diagnosis, my professional experience of working in women's prisons and some of the academic literature.

Anyone who has received the diagnosis of 'BPD' quickly learns of its implicit connection with dangerousness and criminality. A quick Google search reveals stigmatising associations with fictional characters such as Glenn Close, the infamous 'bunny boiler' in the movie *Fatal Attraction*. However, most women who are given this diagnosis are based in the community, where, like me, they are subjected to punitive and blaming treatment, told they are attention-seeking and manipulative, or are simply not seen as legitimately 'mad' enough to warrant support. It is not surprising then that, as psychiatric survivors, we are deeply unhappy with the 'BPD' construct. In a recent consensus statement produced by Lamb and colleagues (2018), most participants indicated that they would like to abandon the term altogether:

> … the label is controversial… it is misleading, stigmatizing and masks the nature of the problem it is supposed to address, adding to the challenges which people experience. (Lamb et al, 2018: 4)

Without further reflection, this process of 'masking' the real problem appears to be some kind of unfortunate and unintended 'side effect' of applying the diagnosis.

However, history has taught us that the psy-professions are far from passively benign in motivation and intention when it comes to the silencing and oppression of women, especially women who have experienced abuse. Cohen (2016: 140) states:

> The history of the psy-professions' pathologisation and abuse of women for being women is deeply disturbing and should shame even the most ardent supporters of the mental health experts. In the name of science and progress, the mental health system has sought to control almost all aspects of women's experiences, emotions, and behaviour through physical and moral interventions.

As a woman who has experienced both sexual violence and the systemic violence brought on by being labelled 'BPD', I believe that there is an ethical imperative to abandon the 'BPD' diagnosis, especially in light of the wider victim-blaming function it is undoubtedly serving.

It is easy to forget that psychiatric diagnoses are merely formulated labels for perceived and sometimes arbitrary clusterings of behaviours. Diagnoses are largely invented by a small section of white, privileged, middle-class, heterosexual men with little to no understanding of what it might be like to be a woman, let alone a woman who has experienced poverty, abuse and violence. As Cohen (2016: 141) elaborates:

> … none of the mental disorders in the DSM with which women have been labelled have validity, psychiatric interventions cannot be argued to be concerned with the care and treatment of any real distress that women may experience. Instead, we need to understand such institutional interventions within the broader context of structural gender inequalities in capitalist society.

This seems like an obvious point to make but it is not one that I remotely considered when told that I had 'borderline personality disorder'. The patriarchal industry of psychiatry has led to the formulation of an astonishing number of diagnoses that blatantly and unapologetically oppress women (Cermele, Daniels & Anderson, 2001). Take, for example, 'female sexual dysfunction'. This diagnosis focuses exclusively on female deficit rather than male surplus and is directly associated with the marketing and sale of female Viagra in the late 1950s (Angel, 2012; Canner, 2008; Caplan & Cosgrove, 2004). In 1987, the proposed inclusion of 'self-defeating personality disorder' ('SDPD') in the revised third edition of the *Diagnostic and Statistical Manual of Mental Disorders (DSM-III-R)* (APA, 1987) positioned victims of domestic and sexual violence as mentally disordered and responsible instigators of their own abuse (Caplan & Gans, 1991; Ritchie, 1989). Even though it was never formally included in the most recent, fifth edition (APA, 2013), the legacy of the proposed construct of 'SDPD' is still extensively seen in clinical judgements and decision-making today (Millon et al, 2012). It is clear that 'personality disorder' has a historical lineage of discrediting and pathologising women's legitimate responses to patriarchal oppression.

'Personality disorder' and imprisoned women

While there has been significant attention and criticism of the 'BPD' diagnosis in community settings (Cahn, 2014; Kinderman, 2015; Kroll, 2003; Langer, 2016; Lewis & Grenyer, 2009; Maidment, 2006; Nyquist-Potter, 2009; Pilgrim, 2001; Samuel & Bucher, 2017), the increasing use of 'personality disorder' diagnoses in forensic settings remains largely unexamined. This is particularly true in the case of 'BPD' and women in such settings: perceived 'symptoms' of the diagnosis (self-injury, displays of 'inappropriate anger' and 'unstable mood') could apply to almost every woman at some point in their forensic journey. Women who receive a 'BPD' diagnosis and women who commit crime, particularly violent crime, appear to share taboo antecedents, such as 'inappropriate and disproportionate anger', 'impulsivity' and a general 'lack of self-control'. Female aggression is an offence to patriarchal-constructed femininity and continues to be pathologised and socially controlled. Some 50–65% of women in prison are believed to meet the criteria for at least one 'personality disorder' (Fazel & Danesh, 2002; Ullrich et al, 2008).

As a woman who has received this diagnosis, it is clear to me that 'BPD' fulfills much of the function that a diagnosis of 'hysteria' might have done in the 1950s: that is, to shut down further enquiry into why women might behave in ways that conflict with societal expectations or might experience extreme periods of distress. The diagnosis also serves to locate the source of distress within a woman's own psyche, removing the need for social responsibility or the scrutiny of oppressive socio-political structures (Gilman et al, 1993). While 'hysteria' as a diagnosis served the function of policing distressed women's conduct, 'BPD' has additional associated 'symptomology' that directly relates to women in the criminal justice system, as Jimenez (1997: 163) explains:

> What distinguishes borderline personality disorder from hysteria is the
> inclusion of anger and other aggressive characteristics, such as shoplifting,
> reckless driving, and substance abuse. If the hysteric was a damaged
> woman, the borderline woman is a dangerous one.

While my experiences of receiving the diagnosis were undoubtedly harmful, it wasn't until I began working in the criminal justice field that I began to realise the full extent of the iatrogenic harm this construct could inflict on women.

Women have a minority status in the criminal justice system. They comprise only five per cent of the total prison population, but they account for 27% of total incidents of self-harm (Ministry of Justice, 2014). Women are much less likely than men to commit violent crime, and the crimes they do commit are frequently under coercion from offending male partners (Barlow, 2015; Jones, 2008; Welle & Falkin, 2000).

Half of all female prisoners report having attempted suicide in their lifetime (Prison Reform Trust, 2017). This is more than twice the rate among male prisoners and more than six times the rate among women in the community (Newcomen, 2017). Since the Corston report (2007),[1] most policy makers now recognise that women are unique as a forensic population, requiring services and support that deal with the multiple, gender-specific disadvantages they have endured. Despite this recognition, women are frequently deprioritised in relation to the larger, more violent male prison population. Prisons are patriarchal structures, historically designed for men, by men, which means that incarcerated women who are facing the prospect of a 'BPD' diagnosis are simultaneously subjected to two patriarchal structures: the psychiatric and the penal.

'Personality disorder' training and the offender 'personality disorder' pathway

I first noticed these dual, intersectional oppressions while working as a trainer and researcher for an expert by experience-led community interest company called Emergence. This was a service-user led organisation that employed anyone with lived experience of being diagnosed with a 'personality disorder'. It initially began by providing coproduction services and arts and social groups based in the community. However, the growing interest and investment in 'personality disorder' within forensic services meant that Emergence could expand and market its services to prisons and forensic mental health units.

---

1. In 2005, the National Reducing Re-offending Delivery Plan outlined seven pathways to reduce re-offending. However, they 'forgot' to include the needs of victims of sexual violence, and it was not until the Corston report (2007), two years later, that two further pathways were added that specifically addressed the unique needs of victims of rape/sexual assault and women who had been victimised by prostitution (Women in Prison, 2017: 12).

Emergence began with noble aspirations to bring about better treatment for those of us who receive a diagnosis of 'personality disorder'. Unfortunately, like many mental health charities, its activism in this arena was curtailed by the reality of having to continually chase contracts for its services, often from the same health organisations responsible for the iatrogenic harm that many of its expert-by-experience employees had survived.

One of Emergence's main sources of income came about as a result of the development of the 'Personality Disorder Capabilities Framework'. The aim of the framework was to empower and educate a workforce so they would be able to work more effectively with people diagnosed with 'personality disorder' and was a direct response to the National Institute for Mental Health in England (NIMHE) report, *Personality Disorder: no longer a diagnosis of exclusion* (NIMHE, 2003). In 2007, following on from recommendations set out in the framework, the Department of Health and the Ministry of Justice commissioned a collaborative partnership between the Institute of Mental Health, the Tavistock and Portman Foundation NHS Trust, the Open University and Emergence. This collaboration saw the development of a nationally operationalised 'personality disorder' educational programme known as the 'Knowledge and Understanding Framework' (KUF).

KUF is the latest attempt to try to change attitudes and behaviour towards those of us who receive a 'personality disorder' diagnosis. Targeting specific populations of professionals, KUF consists of three levels of education: a three-day awareness training package, an undergraduate degree and a master's programme. Since its initial development, KUF has been adapted for delivery in prisons and secure settings, including a gender- specific version called Women's KUF (W-KUF). The training is promoted as innovative and collaborative, with both expert-by-experience trainers and qualified mental health trainers paid at the same rate.

As one of the first-ever expert-by-experience KUF trainers, I felt flattered and valued to be invited to deliver the training alongside qualified psychologists. However, it soon became clear to me that KUF did very little to challenge the validity of the 'BPD' diagnosis, or, indeed, to convey the experiences of service users who had been utterly traumatised by their treatment because of this label. If anything, KUF implicitly defended the legitimacy of the diagnosis, assimilated legitimate trauma narratives into the construct and inadvertently reinforced discrimination-inducing stereotypes. The training incorporated video simulations of actors behaving with child-like emotionality and displaying stereotypically manipulative strategies in order to 'split' staff teams. Expert-by-experience trainers would frequently begin training sessions by uncritically declaring, 'Hello everyone, my name is X and I have narcissistic and borderline personality disorder', followed by a list of their associated *DSM* traits. Nevertheless, since its initial launch, KUF has trained over 30,000 staff members, including those working in female prisons and forensic units.

Alongside the development of KUF arose perhaps one of the most controversial and politically motivated 'personality disorder' diagnoses of all, the government-backed 'dangerous and severe personality disorder' ('DSPD') diagnosis. The 'DSPD' programme consumed excessive amounts of public funding. By 2009 it had cost the public purse £488 million and was known as 'one of the longest running and most expensive pilot programs in UK history' (Rutherford 2010: 46). Despite being evaluated as having failed to achieve any of its aims (O'Loughlin, 2014), in 2011 the 'DSPD' programme was redesigned and expanded into its currently named 'offender personality disorder (OPD) pathway'. Initially designed to 'treat' men who meet the high dangerousness criteria, the OPD pathway was subsequently extended into the female criminal justice context. It now consists of an amalgamation of pre-existing cognitive-based treatments with new transition services called 'psychologically informed planned environments' (PIPEs).

While working as a researcher for Emergence, I interviewed women and prison staff across three prison sites in order to find out what their experiences of 'personality disorder' were and also to explore their views on the potential introduction of the new PIPE service in their prison. Many of the women I spoke with had no idea they had even been given a diagnosis of 'BPD'. Many simply asked if they would get access to improved facilities: 'Will the rooms be any bigger? Can we have cushions? Will I be able to have more visits? Will the officers be nicer over there? Will I get access to some art materials?' I quickly realised that, for most women, simply surviving and improving the immediate prison environment was a main priority. Understandably, incarcerated women would do anything to make their experience of prison more bearable. However, this leaves women extremely vulnerable to having a psy-constructed identity imposed upon them and to accepting the agendas of a coercive prison environment. It is important, then, to question the ethical implications of professionals colonising women's psyches with a profoundly stigmatising and responsibilising[2] identity of 'BPD'.

Later in my career, I worked as a complex case manager at female prison where I witnessed the impact of multiple, confusing discourses surrounding women's 'BPD' diagnosis. These ranged from, 'She's clearly not right in the head,' to 'Well, every woman in here's got that then,' to 'She's not eligible for support because personality disorder is not a real mental illness,' and 'She's just faking it to get something.' Some interventions within the prison involved attempts to convince staff and women that 'BPD' was genetically inherited and should be treated in the same way as any other 'mental illness', both of which are highly contested assumptions. These interventions aimed to combat the high levels of responsibilisation and hostility directed towards incarcerated women with a

---

2. 'Responsibilisation' is a process whereby subjects are rendered individually responsible for a task that previously would have been the duty of another – usually a state agency – or would not have been recognised as a responsibility at all. The process is strongly associated with neoliberal political discourses. (Wakefield & Fleming, 2008).

'BPD' diagnosis. The personality disorder pathway included a series of psycho-educational workshops emphasising this heritability point and at times these workshops felt almost identical to some of the core messages embedded into the KUF training programme.

The emphasis on heritability is not surprising, given the high levels of blame associated with a 'BPD' diagnosis. It is commonly assumed that if 'BPD', like other diagnoses, has associations of 'chemical imbalance' and 'brain disorder' narratives surrounding it, then attitudes towards those of us with the diagnosis would improve. I experienced this while working at Emergence, where there was an idealisation of '*real* mental illness'. I recall a fellow expert-by-experience saying, 'If only they took us as seriously as schizophrenics.' This highlights the way anti-'personality disorder' activism is distinct from other forms of anti-diagnosis activism. Many patients who receive a diagnosis of serious mental illness, such as 'schizophrenia' or 'bipolar disorder', revolt against the infantilisation and intrusive removal of agency that they experience as a result of being diagnosed. In contrast, people with a diagnosis of 'BPD' are not only seen as having complete agency but are over-responsibilised for manifestations of distress and behaviours that are often beyond our capacity to control. Perhaps this is why there is pressure to promote heritability factors in relation to 'BPD'. Unfortunately, as in the case of 'schizophrenia', promoting explanations about brain disorder and illness do not seem to reduce stigma or increase empathic response to those with a diagnosis of 'personality disorder' (Cooke & Kinderman 2018; Corrigan & Watson, 2004).

Clark and colleagues (2015) led a series of psycho-educational workshops in an attempt to promote empathic responding in forensic mental health staff working with patients diagnosed with 'BPD'. The workshops had the sole purpose of promoting the idea that 'BPD' originates from biological and genetic factors. The study found that, despite staff reporting an increase in knowledge regarding 'BPD', they described no difference in empathic response towards the patients in their care. In light of this, it is fair to postulate that so called 'psycho-educational' programmes of this type may sustain oppressive and prejudicial beliefs regarding distressed people, rather than challenge them. Yet psycho-educational workshops for incarcerated women are common and, indeed, form part of the OPD pathway. Like a student at the epistemic mercy of a biased and apolitical teacher, women are presented with uncritical, pseudo-facts about their 'BPD' diagnosis and what they can do in order to take responsibility for their own behaviours and wellbeing. There is no presentation or exploration of the current debates and controversies surrounding the diagnosis. Furthermore, workshops like these are often mandatory for women who are fulfilling the requirements of their sentence plan. Their completion is often used to provide evidence that women have reduced their own 'risk.'

Having examined some of the historical and present-day problems in relation to incarcerated women and 'personality disorder', I am now going to explore some of possible functions 'personality disorder' discourses might serve in forensic contexts.

Why not a trauma pathway?

It is no surprise that incarcerated women have extensive trauma histories (Covington, 2007; Williams, Poyser & Hopkins, 2012). In addition, they are twice as likely to report symptoms consistent with 'PTSD' than their male counterparts (Singleton, Gatward & Meltzer, 1998). Manifestations of distress commonly associated with the diagnosis of 'PTSD' are also more severe in female populations (Sarkar & di Lustro, 2011), and childhood trauma has been implicated as a primary causal factor in offending behaviour in girls (Belknap, 2007). Trauma severity has also been directly linked to the severity and type of offences women commit (Karatzias et al, 2017). There is seemingly widespread existence of trauma in the lives of women who end up in the criminal justice system, yet a kind of nonchalant apathy surrounds this knowledge.

While the OPD pathway has received extortionate amounts of funding, interventions that directly focus on validating and supporting women to cope with their extensive traumatic pasts are rare, especially interventions that directly address childhood sexual abuse, domestic and sexual violence, and sexual exploitation (Women in Prison, 2017). Most of this work is left to underfunded third-sector organisations. These organisations tend to be reliant on short-term contracts and do not have any legitimated power within the prison system. As a result, they can only provide a limited and sometimes inconsistent service.

In 2013, in recognition of the absence of a trauma-informed culture within women's prisons, philanthropist Lady Edwina Grosvenor personally funded a trauma expert, Dr Stephanie Covington, to deliver a systematic, trauma-informed training package to the female prison estate (Covington, 2007). Covington's work included a strongly non-pathologising approach to women's distress, drawing extensively on traumatology and feminist theory. While this intervention appears to directly name and combat many of core difficulties associated with women's distress and offending cycle, it is not integrated into the formal structural of the prison regime in the same way that the OPD pathway is. As it is an independent, external initiative, it has been rolled out entirely unconnected to the 'personality disorder' pathway.

It is important, then, to reflect on why we have a £64 million, publicly funded pathway for 'personality disorder' yet only very poorly and/or sporadically funded interventions that validate and directly address the needs of traumatised women. Menzies' classic paper 'A case-study in the functioning of social systems as a defence against anxiety' (1960) perhaps provides an illuminating insight into the institutionally defensive system. By drawing on this work we can see how prisons, as patriarchal systems and depleted of resources, might collectively seek to alleviate anxiety by locating responsibility and disorder within traumatised women who require considerable amounts of psychological 'containment'. Within this framework, it is understandable that neoliberally aligned interventions and structures that promote self-regulation and emotional control can be implemented without any scrutiny of their socio-political context.

My own research comparing forensic expert perspectives on complex trauma and 'BPD' provides further insight into the possible function of 'personality disorder' ideology in prison contexts (Timoclea & Eaton, in press). One of the main findings was that 'personality disorder' as a construct provided a solution to the cognitive dissonance experienced by many forensic staff and the government departments that fund the prison industrial complex. What is constantly being navigated is the duty of care owed to incarcerated women and the sense that they do not deserve care because they have committed an offence. It seems that the prison system – and, indeed, we as a society – cannot acknowledge the social injustice that many women endured before incarceration. Yet, the horrifying facts about their traumatic lives cannot be erased. To say that a woman's personality is disordered provides a cognitive solution to this discordant reality by acknowledging some 'illness-type' state while simultaneously locating the blame and solution for this 'illness' within the woman.

Incarcerated women are constantly required to navigate forensic staff's cognitive dissonance with regards to their dual victim/perpetrator identities. What ensues is a confusing conglomeration of agency versus infantilisation discourses within the prison environment, and very often within the women themselves. Attempts to acknowledge women's extensive histories of victimisation become assimilated into individualising and responsibilising 'personality disorder' rhetoric, supported by an assortment of behavioural-based interventions which Godsi (2004) refers to as a modern-day, psy equivalent of the witches' dunking stool. A clear example of this is the current trend towards assimilation of the Power, Threat, Meaning Framework (Johnstone & Boyle, 2018) into the 'personality disorder' construct (Willmot & Evershed, 2018).

Some researchers have gone to great lengths to try to maintain the responsibilisation rhetoric surrounding 'BPD' while simultaneously separating it from and cautioning against blame discourse. Pickard (2011), for example, has argued that encouraging us as service users to take responsibility for our self-harm is essential:

> … treatments require clinicians to encourage service users to take responsibility for their behavior, to choose and learn to act otherwise, if they are to improve, let alone recover. (Pickard, 2011: 1)

She draws a theoretical distinction between 'detached' and 'affective' blame, arguing that affective blame is detrimental to service users while detached blame and responsibilisation is appropriate and key to our rehabilitation. She later compares this stance to 'the non-judgmental attitude loving parents show their children' (2011: 1).

While this theoretical distinction is perhaps interesting to an elite group of forensic academics, it is unlikely to translate into any practical change in attitude towards incarcerated women who have a 'BPD' diagnosis. First, it is condescending and entirely incorrect to promote the idea that clinicians should view themselves as compassionate parents, gently coercing their child-like, traumatised patients into taking responsibility for their manifestations of distress. Second, for a multitude of reasons, it is unlikely that prison staff are able to make these kinds of in-depth, philosophical distinctions between conceptualisations of responsibility and blame.

One of the main arguments put forward against using a trauma framework to replace 'BPD' is the idea that not everyone who experiences 'BPD symptomology' has a stereotypical trauma narrative. Likewise, not every woman who experiences abuse and trauma will end up in the criminal justice system. Despite research to support the causal relationship between 'BPD' and childhood trauma (Battle et al, 2004; Ball & Links, 2009), there is a group of women in the community who receive the diagnosis and who do not relate their manifestations of distress to traumatic life experiences (Fossati, Maddedu & Maffei, 1999). However, given the rates of historical trauma and abuse in female forensic populations, this proportion of women is very small. If we took an actuarial[3] approach, as opposed to a purely etiological one, we might ask, what is the probability that a woman who ends up in the criminal justice system with a diagnosis of 'BPD' has experienced extreme trauma and abuse? In approaching the issue from this perspective, it is hard to understand how 'BPD' as a construct can be justifiably retained on behalf of the small minority of women in the general population who receive it and do not identify with traumagenic factors.

Perhaps there are other reasons why 'personality disorder' has attracted increasing amounts of interest and funding in forensic settings. The connection between pharmaceutical industry interest and the increasing prevalence of 'BPD' is not as apparent as it might seem with other diagnoses. This is mainly because medication is viewed as contraindicated for 'BPD' and lacks an evidence base (National Institute for Health and Care Excellence, 2009). However, the economic imperative of the pharmaceutical industry appears to have been replaced by a 'personality disorder' industrial complex. The rise of the 'personality disorder' pathway and the national roll-out of the KUF 'personality disorder' training packages have resulted in a wave of self-declared 'personality disorder experts' claiming specialist knowledge in how to effectively manage and treat this apparently mystifying and unfathomably complex subsection of the female population. The KUF MSc was created partly to enable students to design and

---

3. Actuarialism relates to probability and risk within criminal justice contexts.

pitch the creation of new 'personality disorder' services to commissioners. The likely expansion of the 'personality disorder' pathway into children's services should be of considerable ethical concern to us all.

By way of a conclusion, I propose that declaring that an individual has a 'personality disorder' is a political message, not a clinical one. As Nyquist-Potter (2009: 246) writes:

> One man's identity disturbance is another woman's consciousness-raising, her right not only to choose but to make multiple choices in response to her culture, personal development and life situation.

One man's 'inappropriate anger' is a woman's revolt.

Thus, those of us who wish to resist the 'personality disorder' construct are forced into polemic positions in order to validate our own distressing experiences of the diagnosis. While in other socio-political movements, anger can be a force for political change, within the context of resistance to the 'personality disorder' ideology, it is this very anger that is pathologised and taken as further evidence of the presence of 'personality disorder'. This tautological process of silencing dissent and justifiable anger by the criteria of the construct itself fulfills the perlocutionary function of 'personality disorder'. There is no escape from 'personality disorder'. The construct not only invades our own self-appraisal but forms a toxic film, colouring the perceptions and interpretations of anyone involved in our care or 'rehabilitation'.

I ended up in psychiatric services for multiple reasons. None of them was to do with my personality. Like women who end up in the criminal justice system, I had been let down by multiple institutions that were supposedly designed to help girls like me: girls who are justifiably angry; girls who are beaten, raped, neglected, ignored and then not believed; girls who are told to manage our emotions better, to develop healthier coping mechanisms, to deal with our mistrust of authority – all of this while we as a society elect perpetrators of sexual violence as our politicians and leaders.

We are now faced with a psychiatric system that has few services to support those of us who have had multiple traumatic experiences. Women like me are often excluded from the small number of community mental health trauma services for being 'too complex'. Like women in forensic services, this means we have no choice other than to accept a 'personality-disordered' identity in order to access any kind of support. This is a twisted and unacceptable replication of historical, abusive dynamics. Most of us have learnt that we must endure abuse in order to receive 'care'. Is this a message that we wish to perpetuate?

The absence of trauma pathways or, indeed, a robust evidence base for complex trauma interventions, is directly connected to the masking phenomenon of 'BPD'. For years, the 'BPD' diagnosis has served as a dumping ground to alleviate social responsibility and the state's failure to protect young women and girls. While we continue to frame women's manifestations of distress as evidence of 'personality disorder' pathology, we will collude with a collectively unconscious agenda to deny and suppress the realities of the lives of women who have survived child abuse and sexual violence:

> One consequence of this pathologising agenda, however, is that feminist insights into the different pathways women follow into crime, particularly those characterised by male violence and sexual abuse, are transformed into individualistic and psychologised understandings of criminal women. (Player, 2017: 576)

If female forensic systems are to become more trauma informed, they must consider the traumas they are inflicting on women. These include not only the oppressive prison structure but also the ever-expanding psychiatric and 'personality disorder' industrial complex.

References

American Psychiatric Association (2013). *Diagnostic and Statistical Manual of Mental Disorders* (5th ed). Washington, DC: APA.

American Psychiatric Association (1987). *Diagnostic and Statistical Manual of Mental Disorders* (revised 3rd ed). Washington, DC: APA.

Angel K (2012). Contested psychiatric ontology and feminist critique: 'female sexual dysfunction' and the Diagnostic and Statistical Manual. *History of the Human Sciences 25*(4): 3–24.

Ball JS, Links PS (2009). Borderline personality disorder and childhood trauma: evidence for a causal relationship. *Current Psychiatry Reports 11*(1): 63–68.

Barlow C (2015). Silencing the other: gendered representations of co-accused women offenders. *The Howard Journal of Criminal Justice 54*(5): 469–488.

Battle CL, Shea MT, Johnson DM et al (2004). Childhood maltreatment associated with adult personality disorders: findings from the Collaborative Longitudinal Personality Disorders Study. *Journal of Personality Disorders 18*(2): 193–211.

Belknap J (2007). *The Invisible Woman: gender, crime and justice* (3rd ed). Belmont, CA: Thompson Wadsworth.

Cahn BSK (2014). Borderlines of power: women and borderline personality disorder. *Letters: the Semiannual Newsletter of the Robert Penn Warren Center for the Humanities 22*(2): 1–4. www.vanderbilt.edu/rpw_center/newsletter/Letters_Spring14.pdf

Canner E (2008). Sex, lies and pharmaceuticals: the making of an investigative documentary about female sexual dysfunction. *Feminism & Psychology 18*(4): 488–494.

Caplan PJ, Cosgrove L (2004). *Bias in Psychiatric Diagnosis*. Lanham, MD: Jason Aronson.

Caplan PJ, Gans M (1991). Is there empirical justification for the category of self-defeating personality disorder? *Feminism & Psychology 1*(2): 263–278.

Cermele JA, Daniels S, Anderson KL (2001). Defining normal: constructions of race and gender in the DSM-IV casebook. *Feminism & Psychology 11*(2): 229–247.

Clark CJ, Fox E, Long CG (2015). Can teaching staff about the neurobiological underpinnings of borderline personality disorder instigate attitudinal change? *Journal of Psychiatric Intensive Care 11*(1): 43–51.

Cohen BMZ (2016). *Psychiatric Hegemony: a Marxist theory of mental illness*. London: Palgrave Macmillan.

Cooke A, Kinderman P (2018). 'But what about real mental illnesses?' Alternatives to the disease model approach to 'schizophrenia'. *Journal of Humanistic Psychology 58*(1): 47–71.

Corrigan PW, Watson AC (2004). At issue: stop the stigma: call mental illness a brain disease. *Schizophrenia Bulletin 30*(3): 477–479.

Corston J (2007). *The Corston Report*. London: Home Office.

Covington SS (2007). Women and the criminal justice system. *Women's Health Issues 17*(4): 180–182.

Fazel S, Danesh J (2002). Serious mental disorder in 23,000 prisoners: a systematic review of 62 surveys. *The Lancet 359*(9306): 545–550.

Fossati A, Maddedu F, Maffei C (1999). Borderline personality disorder and childhood sexual abuse: a meta-analytic study. *Journal of Personality Disorders 13*: 268–280.

Gilman SL, King H, Porter R, Rousseau GS, Showalter E (1993). *Hysteria Beyond Freud*. Los Angeles, CA: University of California Press.

Godsi E (2004). *Violence and Society: making sense of madness and badness*. Ross-on-Wye: PCCS Books.

Jimenez MA (1997). Gender and psychiatry: psychiatric conceptions of mental disorders in women, 1960–1994. *Affilia 12*(2): 163.

Johnstone L, Boyle M, with Cromby J, Dillon J, Harper D, Kinderman P, Longden E, Pilgrim D, Read J (2018). *The Power Threat Meaning Framework: towards the identification of patterns in emotional distress, unusual experiences and troubled or troubling behaviour, as an alternative to functional psychiatric diagnosis*. Leicester: British Psychological Society.

Jones S (2008). Partners in crime: a study of the relationship between female offenders and their co-defendants. *Criminology & Criminal Justice 8*(2): 147–164.

Karatzias T, Power K, Woolston C et al (2017). Multiple traumatic experiences, post-traumatic stress disorder and offending behaviour in female prisoners. *Criminal Behaviour and Mental Health 28*(1): 72–84.

Kinderman P (2015). Beyond 'disorder': a psychological model of mental health and well-being. In: Crighton D, Towl G. *Forensic Psychology*. Chichester. John Wiley & Sons (pp291–300).

Kroll J (2003). *PTSD/Borderline in Therapy: finding the balance*. New York, NY: WW Norton & Co.

Lamb N, Sibbald S, Stirzaker A (2018). Shining lights in dark corners of people's lives: reaching consensus for people with complex mental health difficulties who are given a diagnosis of personality disorder. *Criminal Behaviour and Mental Health 28*(1): 1–4.

Langer R (2016). Gender, mental disorder and law at the borderline: complex entanglements of victimization and risk. *Psychiatry, Psychology and Law 23*(1): 69–84.

Lewis KL, Grenyer BF (2009). Borderline personality or complex posttraumatic stress disorder? An update on the controversy. *Harvard Review of Psychiatry 17*(5): 322-328.

Maidment M (2006). 'We're not all that criminal.' *Women & Therapy 29*: 75–96.

Menzies IEP (1960). A case-study in the functioning of social systems as a defence against anxiety: a report on a study of the nursing service of a general hospital. *Human Relations 13*(2): 95–121.

Millon T, Millon CM, Meagher SE, Grossman SD, Ramnath R (2012). *Personality Disorders in Modern Life*. Chichester: John Wiley & Sons.

Ministry of Justice (2014). *A Distinct Approach: a guide to working with women offenders*. London: MoJ.

National Institute for Health and Care Excellence (2009). *Borderline Personality Disorder: recognition and management. Clinical guidance CG78*. London: NICE.

National Institute for Mental Health in England (2003). *Personality Disorder: no longer a diagnosis of exclusion. Policy implementation guidance for the development of services for people with personality disorder*. London/Leeds: NIMHE.

Newcomen N (2017). Self-inflicted deaths among female prisoners. Prison and Probation Ombudsman. *Learning Lessons Bulletin: fatal incidents investigations 13* (March).

Nyquist-Potter N (2009). *Mapping the Edges and the In-Between: a critical analysis of borderline personality disorder*. Oxford: Oxford University Press.

O'Loughlin A (2014). The offender personality disorder pathway: expansion in the face of failure? *The Howard Journal of Crime and Justice 53*(2): 173–192.

Pilgrim D (2001). Disordered personalities and disordered concepts. *Journal of Mental Health 10*(3): 253–265.

Player E (2017). The offender personality disorder pathway and its implications for women prisoners in England and Wales. *Punishment & Society 19*(5): 568–589.

Pickard H (2011). Responsibility without blame: empathy and the effective treatment of personality disorder. *Philosophy, Psychiatry & Psychology 18*(3): 209–223.

Prison Reform Trust (2017). *Prison: the facts*. Bromley Briefings. London: Prison Reform Trust.

Ritchie K (1989). The little woman meets son of DSM-III. *The Journal of Medicine and Philosophy 14*(6): 695–708.

Rutherford M (2010). *Blurring the Boundaries: the convergence of mental health and criminal justice policy, legislation, systems and practice*. London: Sainsbury Centre for Mental Health.

Samuel DB, Bucher MA (2017). Assessing the assessors: the feasibility and validity of clinicians as a source for personality disorder research. *Personality Disorders: Theory, Research, and Treatment 8*(2): 104–112.

Sarkar J, di Lustro M (2011). Evolution of secure services for women in England. *Advances in Psychiatric Treatment 17*(5): 323–331.

Singleton N, Gatward R, Meltzer H (1998). *Psychiatric Morbidity Among Prisoners in England and Wales*. London: Stationery Office.

Timoclea R, Eaton J (ed) (in press). *'Demonic Little Mini-Skirted Machiavellis': expert conceptualisations of complex post traumatic stress disorder and borderline personality disorder in female forensic populations*. VictimFocus Publications.

Ullrich S, Deasy D, Smith J et al (2008). Detecting personality disorders in the prison population of England and Wales: comparing case identification using the SCID-II screen and the SCID-II clinical interview. *The Journal of Forensic Psychiatry & Psychology 19*(3): 301–322.

Wakefield A, Fleming J (eds) (2008). *The Sage Dictionary of Policing*. London: Sage Publications Ltd.

Williams K, Poyser J, Hopkins K (2012). *Accommodation, Homelessness and Reoffending of Prisoners: results from the Surveying Prisoner Crime Reduction (SPCR) survey*. London: Ministry of Justice.

Willmot P, Evershed S (2018). Interviewing people given a diagnosis of personality disorder in forensic settings. *International Journal of Forensic Mental Health 17*(4): 338–350.

Welle D, Falkin G (2000). The everyday policing of women with romantic codefendants: an ethnographic perspective. *Women & Criminal Justice 11*(2): 45–65.

Women in Prison (2017). *Corston 10+: the Corston Report 10 years on*. London: Women in Prison. www.womeninprison.org.uk/perch/resources/corston-report-10-years-on.pdf (accessed 22 November 2017).

12 | Working therapeutically with clients with a psychiatric diagnosis

Terry Lynch

Often referred to as the bible of psychiatry, the *Diagnostic and Statistical Manual of Mental Disorders* (American Psychiatric Association (APA), 2013) and its European equivalent, the *International Classification of Diseases* (World Health Organization, 2018), are widely accepted as the definitive diagnostic references in relation to 'mental disorders'.

The American Psychiatric Association (APA) – the creator and publisher of the *DSM* – refers to it as 'the authoritative guide to the diagnosis of mental disorders' (American Psychiatric Association, undated-a). With a few notable exceptions, within the disciplines of psychology, psychotherapy, counselling and most other mental health professions, the *DSM* is similarly viewed as the most authoritative reference in relation to the psychiatric diagnoses. In considering the issue of counsellors, psychotherapists, psychologists, social workers and other mental health disciplines working therapeutically with people who have been given a psychiatric diagnosis, an important first step is becoming aware of some important facts in relation to the *DSM*.

Given the high level of authority bestowed upon the *DSM*, one might reasonably expect that its validity has been thoroughly established. Counter-intuitive though it might seem, this is not the case.

Perhaps because the creators of the *DSM* were medical doctors, members of one of the most trusted professions in the world, the media and public alike assumed that, as the APA and its task force heads increasingly claimed, it was scientific and must be grounded on a solid, scientific evidence base, giving it a high level of validity.

In fact, the validity of the *DSM* is poles apart from the exalted authority with which it is held. Even within mainstream psychiatry, serious questions regarding its validity have been raised since the publication of *DSM-III* (APA, 1980). For example, prominent American psychiatrist Nancy Andreasen has written that, in creating this third edition, 'validity has been sacrificed to achieve reliability' and '*DSM* diagnoses are not useful for research because of their lack of validity' (Andreasen, 2007). Former director of the American National Institute of Mental Health, Thomas Insel has similarly said of the *DSM* that 'the weakness is its lack of validity' (Insel, 2013).

If the *DSM* diagnoses are not useful for research due to lack of validity, surely their usefulness in other considerations is inevitably similarly compromised? Elsewhere, Thomas Insel, commenting on the lack of any meaningful biological content within the *DSM*, has remarked that 'biology never read that book' (Belluck & Carey, 2013). Maria Angell – a former editor-in-chief of the *New England Journal of Medicine* and senior lecturer at the Department of Global Health & Social Medicine at Harvard Medical School – has written that:

> Given its importance, you might think that the *DSM* represents the authoritative distillation of a large body of scientific evidence. It is instead the product of a complex of academic politics, personal ambition, ideology and, perhaps most important, the influence of the pharmaceutical industry. What the *DSM* lacks is evidence.
>
> The problem with the *DSM* is that in all of its editions it has simply reflected the opinions of its writers. Not only did the *DSM* become the bible of psychiatry, but like the real Bible, it depends on something akin to revelation. There are no citations of scientific studies to support its decisions. That is an astonishing omission, because in all medical publications, whether journals or books, statements of fact are supposed to be supported by citations of scientific studies. (Angell, 2009)

The *DSM* has no scientific validity. There is no scientific basis to the *DSM*. It is the product of consensus, not science.

The validity of the concept of mental disorder

The importance of the notion of so-called mental disorders to those who promote the prevailing medical approach to mental health is reflected in the inclusion of this term in the *DSM* title – *The Diagnostic and Statistical Manual of Mental Disorders*. Remarkably, according to the medical profession, 50% of the population will have a 'mental disorder' during their lifetime (Rosenberg, 2013).

The entire basis upon which 21st century psychiatry is built is dependent on the continuing widespread public acceptance of the validity of the concept of 'mental disorder'. To a large extent, mainstream psychiatrists have persuaded themselves, other mental health professionals and the public that 'mental disorders' are real entities, real brain disorders, real medical illnesses.

This premise is incorrect. The experiences and behaviours that come to be grouped as various psychiatric diagnoses are in themselves real and entirely valid. The extrapolation that these experiences and behaviours constitute real medical illnesses, real medical entities, has no scientific foundation.

Inadequacy of training of mental health professionals

Spearheaded by the almost universal erroneous belief in the validity of the *DSM* and the legitimacy of the concept of so-called mental disorders, the prevailing view of the experiences and behaviours that come to be diagnosed as 'mental disorders' assumes the presence of biological abnormalities. However, this has little or no corresponding scientific verification. This false understanding has resulted in the minimisation of the relevance of many aspects of the experiences and behaviours described as 'mental disorders'.

An important consequence of the long-standing systematic medicalisation of human distress has been a diminished focus on the psychiatric diagnoses within training programmes for non-medical mental health professionals. Many psychology, psychotherapy and counselling training courses have mistakenly accepted the much-promoted but incorrect notion that 'mental disorders' are scientifically verified medical illnesses, best dealt with from a predominantly medical perspective.

Consequently, non-medical mental health professionals generally receive inadequate training in relation to the psychiatric diagnoses. The little training that such trainees receive tends to largely accept the medical model, rather than explore the emotional and psychological aspects of the experiences and behaviours that come to be diagnosed as 'mental illnesses'. This is a great shame; counselling, psychotherapy and psychology have the potential to play a far more significant role in relation to the psychiatric diagnoses than they do.

A recovery-oriented mental health service

Since 2001, I have provided a recovery-oriented mental health service. The majority of the people who consult me have previously received a psychiatric diagnosis. I have accumulated 17 years of first-hand experience of working with people who had been given various psychiatric diagnoses, including 'depression', 'general anxiety disorder', 'bipolar disorder', 'obsessive compulsive disorder', 'schizophrenia', 'personality disorders', 'eating disorders' and 'schizo-affective disorder'. The recovery rates in my service are far higher than typically occurs within the mental health services. For the past two years, I have created courses to help mental health professionals understand psychiatric diagnoses from a more psychologically focused approach.

For 10 years prior to setting up this recovery-oriented mental health service, I worked as a general practitioner. In the latter years of this work, I became increasingly concerned about the medical approach to mental health. During those years, my progressive questioning of the prevailing approach to mental health centred on three themes: my increasing awareness of a) the paucity of solid evidence base of biological pathology within psychiatry compared with all other branches of medicine, despite regular claims to the contrary; b) the gross underestimation of the emotional and psychological characteristics of people's experiences and behaviours, and c) how helpful interventions with primarily emotional, psychological and social components often were, which would not be the case if psychiatry's claims of the primacy of biology in mental health were correct.

All experiences and behaviours are purposeful

All of the experiences and behaviours that come to be diagnosed as various mental illnesses are purposeful in some way. This truth forms the platform for a far richer understanding of these experiences and behaviours, laying the foundation for a coherent and credible recovery-oriented approach.

The medicalisation of human distress has been an integral factor in the growth of public acceptance of the concept of mental illness – an acceptance based on the erroneous belief that the medicalisation of distress was grounded upon a solid, verified evidence base.

A regrettable consequence of the progressive medicalisation of human distress has been the disregarding of anything approaching an adequate commitment to deepening the understanding of possible emotional and psychological components of psychiatric diagnoses. The widespread but mistaken acceptance of the *DSM* as a valid, scientifically grounded reference guide has contributed greatly to this deplorable situation. As American psychiatrist Daniel Carlat has written, the *DSM* 'has drained the color out of the way we understand and treat our patients. It has de-emphasized psychological-mindedness, and replaced it with the illusion that we understand our patients when all we are doing is assigning them labels' (Carlat, 2010: 60).

The de-emphasising of psychological-mindedness to which Daniel Carlat refers is at the root of the failure of the prevailing mental health approach to make a significant impact on global mental health. As a member and a keen observer of the medical profession for more than 30 years, I believe the gross lack of interest in the psychology of the psychiatric diagnoses is no coincidence; it serves to reinforce the position of the medical profession at the top of the global mental health pyramid of expertise. Although unjustified in terms of its actual rather than perceived expertise, this position of primacy yields major benefits for the medical profession in terms of status, importance and power in global mental health. If we are to work therapeutically with people who have been given psychiatric diagnoses, we have to correct this distorted approach. What is needed is a paradigm shift.

This endemic lack of psychological-mindedness surfaces regularly within mainstream mental health services, greatly impeding the potential for people to live happier and more fulfilled lives. People diagnosed with psychiatric diagnoses such as 'bipolar disorder', 'schizophrenia', 'personality disorder' and, in many cases, 'depression', 'OCD' and other psychiatric diagnoses, are often told by their doctors that there is no cure, that the best they can hope for is long-term maintenance treatment with medication. Such assertions often originate from supposedly authoritative sources.

For example, according to the American National Institute of Mental Health: 'Right now, there is no cure for bipolar disorder' (National Institute of Mental Health, undated-a). This is false information. I personally know more than three dozen people who have made an excellent recovery from a legitimate diagnosis of 'bipolar disorder', and many who have made an excellent recovery having been given a legitimate diagnosis of 'schizophrenia'. By 'legitimate' I mean meeting the medical criteria for these diagnoses.

On hearing stories of full recovery from diagnoses such as 'bipolar disorder' and 'schizophrenia', a typical reaction of psychiatrists and GPs is to state that it must have been a misdiagnosis; that the person could not have had 'bipolar disorder' to begin with, since recovery from 'bipolar disorder' does not happen, according to the medical ideology. The fundamental ideologies and tenets of psychiatry are thus preserved, including the false claim that such psychiatric diagnoses are medical illnesses, just like diabetes. The people to whom I refer as having made excellent recoveries met the psychiatric criteria for these diagnoses. By psychiatry's own standards, therefore, they were legitimate diagnoses.

For mental health professionals to work more effectively with people who have been given a psychiatric diagnosis, a greater understanding of the person's inner world is a prerequisite. This is generally a routine and much-valued aspect of counselling and psychotherapy, but prioritising the understanding of people's inner worlds has been greatly limited by psychiatry's pathologisation and medicalisation of such experiences. This results in bypassing due consideration of the person's inner world. This is a great mistake.

A wounding-to-resolution cycle

I have found the following to be a helpful aid in understanding the origin of the experiences and behaviours that subsequently become diagnosed as various so-called mental illnesses and a pathway through which they develop.

According to American psychotherapist Virginia Satir:

> By the time we reach the age of five, we probably have had a billion experiences in sharing communication. By that age we have developed

> ideas about how we see ourselves, what we can expect from others, and
> what seems to be possible or impossible for us in the world. (Satir, 1988: 52)

A key point is not whether Satir's figure of one billion experiences is accurate, but that, by the age of five, a child has had an enormous number of interactions. Through these experiences and interactions – and the child's own personal experience and interpretation of these interactions – they are developing their perception of themselves in relation to others and the world. As the child continues through the remainder of their childhood, into and through the teenage years and into their 20s, they continue this ongoing process of self-perception and self-evaluation in relation to others, the world, how best to interact with the world, how best to get their needs met, what seems possible and not possible for them, and other relevant priorities.

It is inevitable that some interactions will be experienced adversely, as woundings. What matters is the overall accumulation of these interactions, as experienced by the individual, their impact, and the conclusions arrived at by the individual in relation to how they see and experience themselves in the world.

Wounding is a common forerunner to the development of the experiences and behaviours that subsequently become diagnosed as various psychiatric 'illnesses'. Varying degrees and states of woundedness are frequently present within people who have been given a psychiatric diagnosis. Wounding is commonly followed by *shock*, a state characterised by disbelief, denial, confusion, difficulty concentrating, being easily startled and other experiences and behaviours, all of which are common features of many so-called mental illnesses. States of shock may continue long after the wounding is experienced.

Distress regularly follows wounding and shock. Distress can be experienced in many forms, such as hurt, loss, overwhelm, anger, anxiety, sadness, tears, aloneness, grief, rejection and abandonment. Depending on the level of distress and the degree to which the child's environment meets their needs, the emerging child may resort to some of the many possible *defence mechanisms* and *coping strategies*.

If the emerging child's environment supports the experiencing and expression of distress in a healthy and balanced fashion, the child learns to feel their feelings, trust in them, express them and bring them through to resolution of the distress and any related needs. If the emerging child's environment does not support the experiencing and expression of their emotions and their needs, the child may resort to various defence mechanisms and coping strategies in an attempt to get by.

Recently, a female client in her mid-20s recalled a moment from her school years, when she was seven years of age. A child of similar age fell in the schoolyard, hurting their knee. The child began to cry loudly. She recalled looking at this child with surprise, wondering why the child would bother crying, since crying never achieved anything. By the age of seven, she had already concluded that there was no point in crying. She had stopped crying years earlier. It emerged that circumstances within her home were such that there was little support for her emotional state and her needs. Living in such an environment, as a coping strategy, she learned to suppress much of herself, including many of her emotions and her needs.

It is not uncommon for such children to become diagnosed with a so-called mental illness later in life. This young woman was diagnosed with 'clinical depression' in her late teens. The experiences and behaviours that resulted in her being diagnosed with 'depression' were eminently understandable from the standpoint of wounding, shock, distress, defence mechanisms/coping strategies, choice and patterns of choice-making, and trauma. From a recovery perspective, this latter way of understanding is far more accurate than the prevailing unverified belief in brain abnormalities and genetics.

Making sense of 'anhedonia'

Each of the nine criteria for a diagnosis of 'depression' can be far better understood from a psychological standpoint than from a concocted biological perspective for which there is little or no evidence base. To illustrate this, I will now discuss one of the nine 'depression' criteria: 'anhedonia' – the loss of interest in pleasurable activities, no longer feeling pleasure in activities generally considered pleasurable.

Within the prevailing understanding of mental health, anhedonia has long been viewed as a biological and core feature of so-called clinical depression. No biological, pathological abnormalities have yet been reliably linked to 'anhedonia', yet the medical assumption of biological causation continues to dominate discussions about it. From a psychological perspective, however, 'anhedonia' can be thoroughly understood. In people who reach the point of not being able to experience pleasure, there is generally a story, a journey they have undertaken in the years prior to the identification of emotional and mental health problems.

The woman I mentioned above is a typical example. Her GP and psychiatrists assumed a fundamental biological basis to her stated condition, which included her being unable to experience pleasure.

In her work with me, it became clear that, from a young age, she developed a range of defence mechanisms and coping strategies in an attempt to get by, to survive. Living within a family environment that was not conducive to the expression of emotions and the meeting of her needs, she learned to suppress both her emotions and her needs to the greatest degree possible.

Like many things in life, defence mechanisms and coping strategies can be a double-edged sword. If I break my leg, I am likely to need crutches for a few weeks. If I use the crutches for the optimal time and cease using them when I am ready to progress without them, the crutches will have served me well. There will be no ongoing repercussions. What if I decide to continue using my crutches for a further two years, because I feel safe and secure when using them? In such a scenario, I have chosen to prioritise the feelings of safety and security inherent in the ongoing use of crutches, perhaps including a sense of safety and security that having limits apparently imposed outside my control may provide.

We create our defence mechanisms and coping strategies for understandable reasons. For my female client, such major degrees of suppression of emotion can be the lesser of two evils in comparison with the disappointment and heartbreak of expressing emotions and needs to important people in her life and not having these emotions and needs honoured and met. Hence her surprise at seeing a fellow schoolchild crying, having hurt their knee.

Such defence mechanisms are protective and understandable. However, as with the crutches scenario, continued maintenance of defence mechanisms and coping strategies long after the initial need invited their creation often results in a whole series of other problems. Having resorted to the suppression of her emotions and needs in her early childhood, this young woman came to trust in this way of operating in the world. Suppression became all she knew and trusted, so, through her late teens and 20s, she continued this pattern.

As a general rule, there are consequences for actions and choices. Having committed to suppressing the experiencing and expression of emotions such as hurt and sorrow, she rendered other experiences and emotions, such as happiness and joy, unattainable. You cannot block access to some core primary emotions and have free access to others; block some core primary emotions, and you risk blocking them all. If, over many years, I have become practised at numbing hurt, sorrow, sadness and loss, I will also need to have numbed any possibility of feeling joy. Allowing myself to fully feel joy would result in my letting go of the subtle but high level of vigilance I have put in place to ensure I do not feel my long-held sorrow, losses and grief. If I have long since decided that a main priority is to ensure that I do not come into full emotional contact with my accumulated sorrow, woundedness and trauma, then suppressing joy and pleasure will likely be a price I am willing to pay.

This constitutes a far more viable explanation for 'anhedonia' than that provided by fanciful claims of biological brain abnormalities – claims that remain unverified, despite 70 years of intense research aimed at establishing a biological bedrock for emotional and psychological problems. Not feeling pleasure is the price paid for prioritising the perceived need to continue blocking the full feeling and expression of wounding, distress and trauma.

Reduced selfhood

Links between reduced self-esteem and psychiatric diagnoses have long been observed. For example, the authors of a 2003 study noted: 'Much previous research indicates that lowered self-esteem frequently accompanies psychiatric disorders' (Silverstone & Salsali, 2003). The contrast between the medical enthusiasm to research biologically-related possibilities, such as brain chemical imbalances and genetics, and psychologically-related possibilities, such as low self-esteem, is striking. This is no accident: thoroughly researching self-esteem and applying considerations of self-esteem in a meaningful way to psychiatric diagnoses would likely increase the focus on the psychological aspects of the experiences and behaviours that come to be so diagnosed. This would risk dislodging biology as the key aspect of the psychiatric diagnoses and, with it, the primacy of the medical profession's status as *the* global mental health experts.

While relevant, the concept of self-esteem as an individual's sense of his or her own value or worth (Blascovich & Tomaka, 1991) is insufficient to encapsulate the degree to which many aspects of the self can become compromised. This is also true in relation to people who receive a psychiatric diagnosis. I have therefore set out a more expanded description of relevant aspects of self in my book *Selfhood* (Lynch, 2011). In this book, I describe many aspects of the self that are regularly compromised in people given a psychiatric diagnosis, including boundaries and personal space; self-belonging; self-expression; self-empowerment; self-generated security; comfort zones; self-care; self-contact; self-regulation; dealing with emotions; needs, and need-meeting. As was the case in relation to my female client at seven years of age, the process of self-compromisation typically begins years before the diagnosis, often gradually increasing in intensity in the years prior to being diagnosed. I refer to this as self-compromisation because it is the individual who orchestrates the compromise in response to their particular interpretation of their experiences in life.

None of the much-vaunted references to brain chemical imbalances, other putative brain problems and genetic abnormalities are demonstrable in any person who has been given any psychiatric diagnosis. Nor do they play any meaningful role in the day-to-day management of any psychiatric diagnosis. In contrast, the aspects I describe in this chapter are commonly present and can be worked with, both in therapy and by the person themselves, with appropriate support and guidance.

Agency, self-empowerment and self-efficacy

Agency is 'the state of being in action or exerting power' (Definitions, undated). Self-empowerment can be defined as 'taking control of our own life, setting goals, and making positive choices' (Shah, 2015). Self-efficacy refers to 'a person's belief about his or her ability and capacity to accomplish a task or to deal with the challenges of life' (BusinessDictionary, undated). Referring to self-efficacy as 'people's beliefs about their capabilities to produce designated levels of performance that exercise influence over events that affect their lives', Bandura (1994) states: 'Self-efficacy beliefs determine how people feel, think, motivate themselves and behave.'

The importance of these interlinking themes to emotional and mental health cannot be overstated. Yet, because of the dominance of the biologically biased medical model of mental health, these themes do not receive anything approaching a commensurate degree of attention in relation to the psychiatric diagnoses. This oversight is most regrettable, given that issues relating to agency, self-empowerment and self-efficacy are closely linked to each of the main psychiatric diagnoses.

Experience gained through working full-time in a psychotherapeutic recovery-oriented fashion for 17 years with people given psychiatric diagnoses has enabled me to identify that a greatly reduced perceived sense of agency, self-empowerment and self-efficacy are key elements within people who are diagnosed with 'schizophrenia', 'bipolar disorder', 'personality disorder', 'obsessive compulsive disorder', 'eating disorders', 'depression' and 'general anxiety disorder'. I have generally found that people given a diagnosis of 'schizophrenia' tend to have the greatest degree of loss of agency, self-empowerment and self-efficacy. While there can be a greater degree of variation of these losses in relation to the other psychiatric diagnoses, a noticeable degree of loss in relation to these three themes is almost always present.

As a general rule, non-medical mental health disciplines are far more attuned to the importance of working directly with issues relating to agency, self-empowerment and self-efficacy than medical doctors who work in mental health, such as psychiatrists and GPs. In my 30 years of medical practice, during which I have had ongoing contact both with people attending mental health services and mental health services themselves, I could count on one hand the number of occasions where agency, self-empowerment or self-efficacy was recognised and addressed to any degree, and still have several fingers to spare.

The medical radar is set to pick up what the medical ideology prioritises. Born primarily out of self- and group-interest and propagation rather than the public interest, the medical ideology wrongly places little value or relevance on possibilities that might diminish its own status and position at the top of the global mental health pyramid of expertise. This is why issues that are obviously present within people who are given a psychiatric diagnosis – issues such as reduced agency, self-empowerment and self-efficacy – are largely airbrushed out of medical considerations regarding what is wrong and what might help.

Trauma

Another such issue is trauma. For decades, the role and relevance of trauma to psychiatric diagnoses have been systematically underestimated and minimised to such a degree that recognised trauma expert, psychiatrist Bessel van der Kolk, has created a presentation entitled 'Psychiatry must stop ignoring trauma' (van der Kolk, 2015).

The grossly distorted approach to trauma adopted by the medical profession is evidenced by the fact that so-called post-traumatic stress disorder

(PTSD) is the only medical diagnosis I know of where what happened defines what is wrong.

According to the UK's National Health Service (NHS): 'Post-traumatic stress disorder (PTSD) can develop after a very stressful, frightening or distressing event, or after a prolonged traumatic experience' (NHS, undated); not just a stressful, frightening or distressing event or traumatic experience, but a *very* stressful frightening or distressing event; not just a traumatic experience, but a *prolonged* traumatic experience. The authors do not appear to have noticed an obvious contradiction within their words; if not all traumatic experiences can cause trauma, why call them traumatic experiences?

The American Psychiatric Association lists the types of experiences necessary for a diagnosis of 'PTSD' to be considered appropriate:

> Posttraumatic Stress Disorder (PTSD) is a psychiatric disorder that can occur in people who have experienced or witnessed a traumatic event such as a natural disaster, a serious accident, a terrorist act, war/combat, rape or other violent personal assault. (American Psychiatric Association, undated-b)

The NHS lists 'the type of events that can lead to PTSD' as:

> … serious road accidents; violent personal assaults, such as sexual assault, mugging or robbery; prolonged sexual abuse, violence or severe neglect; witnessing violent deaths; military combat; being held hostage; terrorist attacks; natural disasters, such as severe floods, earthquakes or tsunamis; a diagnosis of a life-threatening condition; an unexpected severe injury or death of a close family member or friend. (NHS, undated)

It informs the public that 'PTSD isn't usually related to situations that are simply upsetting, such as divorce, job loss or failing exams' (NHS, undated). I'm not convinced that the vast majority of people who have gone through a divorce, lost their job or failed exams would agree that such experiences are 'simply upsetting'.

This linking of trauma to the type of events that occur is unique within standard medical practice. Finding out what happened to a person is a regular part of a doctor's medical evaluation, but as a general rule doctors do not base their conclusions about what is wrong on what happened to the person. For example, every doctor working in casualty departments knows that fractures can occur as a result of a wide spectrum of events, ranging from major accidents to tripping over the cat. Imagine the chaos – including significant numbers of missed fractures – that would ensue in casualty departments everywhere if the policy regarding fracture assessment was that only people who had experienced major accidents or incidents would be deemed worthy of further fracture assessment, including x-rays.

Raising the bar so high in relation to who qualifies for a diagnosis of 'PTSD' carries significant benefits for mainstream psychiatry. 'PTSD' – and, consequently, trauma – is thus relegated in importance and frequency as a relatively rare situation caused by major incidents that are not commonly experienced. Psychiatry has instead focused more on supposed 'mental illnesses' that fit more comfortably into its own ideology. For example, in contrast to the uncommon preconditions attached to a diagnosis of 'PTSD', 'depression can strike at any time' (APA, undated-c).

In 2017 I was an invited speaker at a training day attended by more than 100 GPs. I asked for a show of hands on which of two so-called psychiatric diagnoses they felt more familiar, comfortable and confident with: 'PTSD' or 'depression'. Every single GP in the room raised their hand in favour of 'depression'. The vast majority of psychiatric diagnoses are made by GPs, whose training in mental health often leaves much to be desired. Being human, GPs (and psychiatrists) are likely to gravitate towards practices – such as diagnosing and prescribing – with which they feel comfortable and confident. This reality goes some way towards explaining the relentless rise in the rates of both the diagnosis of 'depression' and antidepressant prescribing – 64.7 million prescriptions were given out in 2016 in England alone, more than its entire population (Campbell, 2017).

Regrettably, this approach to trauma has filtered into the world of psychology. The American Psychological Association defines trauma as 'an emotional response to a terrible event like an accident, rape or natural disaster' (American Psychological Association, undated-d). According to this definition, an event must be at the level of 'terrible' for trauma to have considered to have occurred.

This prevailing approach to trauma fails to take into account the reality that wounding and trauma are relatively common occurrences in life. Wounding, trauma and their effects are frequent components of the experiences and behaviours than come to be diagnosed as various so-called mental illnesses. Rather than erroneously being seen as occurring and being outside the range of normal human experience, trauma needs to be seen for what it is – a commonly occurring phenomenon, personal to the individual.

'Paranoia'

In definitions and considerations of 'paranoia', the word 'unreasonable' regularly appears. For example, the Cambridge Dictionary defines 'paranoia' as 'an extreme and unreasonable feeling that other people do not like you or are going to harm or criticize you'. In keeping with the general understanding of the term, the Cambridge Dictionary also states: 'Someone who has paranoia has unreasonable false beliefs as a part of another mental illness, for example schizophrenia' (Cambridge Dictionary, undated).

This common understanding fails to capture the essence of the experiences and behaviours that become described as 'paranoia'. Understanding 'paranoia' requires an understanding of the inner world of the person. Common themes are inner convictions of being powerless in the world; feeling unsafe and being unable to make oneself feel safe in many situations; considerable woundedness and a consequent fear/terror of being further wounded; a conviction that one cannot cope. A person with such an experiential inner world may unconsciously project these feelings onto the screen of life, seeing and feeling danger in situations where others would not have such feelings. These are not 'unreasonable' feelings, experiences and behaviours; they are entirely reasonable from the person's standpoint. Understanding this is a first step towards working therapeutically with people who have such experiences.

'Delusions'

'Delusions' are variously defined and described as 'beliefs that have no basis in reality' (National Institute of Mental Health, undated-b); 'very strong beliefs which are obviously untrue to others, but not to you' (Royal College of Psychiatrists, undated) and 'a false belief that is based on an incorrect interpretation of reality' (Harvard Health Publishing, 2012). We are told, 'a person with a delusion will hold firmly to the belief regardless of evidence to the contrary' (Kiran & Chaudhury, 2009).

Within the prevailing view of mental health, beliefs that come to be understood as 'delusions' are taken as evidence of serious mental illness such as 'schizophrenia'. Within this prevailing view, it is assumed that there is little point in seeking to understand or make sense of such beliefs. Once they are deemed as having no basis in reality and that they continue to be held with conviction despite the person being presented with evidence of the belief being false, doctors generally feel that there is no point in any further exploration. It is assumed that 'delusions' are so bizarre that they must constitute evidence of serious mental illness. The typical medical response is to prescribe antipsychotic medication, a primary action of which is usually sedation.

By taking the person's inner world into account, one can arrive at a far richer and more accurate understanding of these beliefs. Many so-called delusions represent the externalisation or projection of a deeply held need or fear. For example, people who become convinced that they are a singularly important person or that they have special powers typically have had a very low sense of self-worth for some time. Seeking to convince themselves and others that they are extremely important is an attempt to compensate for their long-felt sense of unimportance. In my work, I have often found that working with people's sense of self and self-empowerment can help develop a self-perception within which there is more empowerment and so less need for the so-called delusion.

Where fear is a trigger for a delusion, there is usually an accompanying sense of powerlessness, within which the person regularly feels unsafe, under threat, and incapable of ameliorating their situation or making generating safety from within themselves.

Conclusion

Given the lack of validity of the *DSM* and the serious questions surrounding the legitimacy of the concept of mental disorder, a reappraisal of both the nature of emotional and mental health problems and the potential role of mental health practitioners of various disciplines is appropriate, necessary and in the public interest.

Psychiatry is the only area of medicine that does not routinely aim for the best possible and available outcomes; maintenance rather than recovery is its primary focus. In the public interest, this must change. Also in the public interest, it behoves the non-medical mental health disciplines to take a more central place in relation to the psychiatric diagnoses and those who find themselves being given such diagnoses. To paraphrase Edmund Burke's adage, 'The only thing necessary for evil to thrive is for good men to do nothing.' The failure of the non-medical mental health disciplines to take a stand in relation to the psychiatric diagnoses has contributed in no small way to the unjustified dominance of a biologically biased approach to global mental health that is scientifically unverified and largely devoid of anything approaching an adequate psychological understanding.

References

American Psychiatric Association (2013). *Diagnostic and Statistical Manual of Mental Disorders* (5th ed). Washington: American Psychiatric Association.

American Psychiatric Association (1980). *Diagnostic and Statistical Manual of Mental Disorders* (3rd ed). Washington: American Psychiatric Association.

American Psychiatric Association (undated-a). *Frequently asked questions.* [Online.] www.psychiatry.org/psychiatrists/practice/dsm/feedback-and-questions/frequently-asked-questions (Accessed 4 April 2018).

American Psychiatric Association (undated-b). *Help with posttraumatic stress disorder (PTSD).* [Online.] www.psychiatry.org/patients-families/ptsd (accessed 18 April 2018).

American Psychiatric Association (undated-c). *What is depression?* [Online.] (www.psychiatry.org/patients-families/depression/what-is-depression (accessed 12 June 2019).

American Psychological Association (undated-d). *Trauma.* [Online]. www.apa.org/topics/trauma/ (accessed 18 April 2018).

Andreasen N (2007). DSM and the death of phenomenology in America: an example of unintended consequences. *Schizophrenia Bulletin 33*(1): 108–112.

Angell M (2009). Drug companies and doctors: a story of corruption. [Online.] *New York Review of Books*; 15 January. www.nybooks.com/articles/2009/01/15/drug-companies-doctorsa-story-of-corruption/ (accessed 10 April 2017).

Bandura A (1994). Self-efficacy. In: Ramachaudran VS (ed). *Encyclopedia of Human Behavior* Vol 4. New York: Academic Press (pp71–81). (Reprinted in: Friedman H (ed) (1998). *Encyclopedia of Mental Health*. San Diego: Academic Press.)

Belluck P, Carey B (2013). Psychiatry's guide is out of touch with science, experts say. *New York Times*; 6 May. www.nytimes.com/2013/05/07/health/psychiatrys-new-guide-falls-short-experts-say.html (accessed 12 April 2017).

Blascovich J, Tomaka J (1991). Measures of self-esteem. In: Robinson JP, Shaver PR, Wrightsman LS (eds). *Measures of Personality and Social Psychological Attitudes, Volume I*. San Diego, CA: Academic Press.

BusinessDictionary (undated). *Self-efficacy*. www.businessdictionary.com/definition/self-efficacy.html (accessed 16 April 2018).

Cambridge Dictionary (undated). *Paranoia*. https://dictionary.cambridge.org/dictionary/english/paranoia (accessed 17 April 2018).

Campbell D (2017). NHS prescribed record number of antidepressants last year. *The Guardian*; 29 June. www.theguardian.com/society/2017/jun/29/nhs-prescribed-record-number-of-antidepressants-last-year (accessed 19 April 2018).

Carlat, D (2010). *Unhinged: the trouble with psychiatry – a doctor's revelations about a profession in crisis*. London: Free Press.

Definitions (undated). '*Agency*'. www.definitions.net/definition/agency (accessed 16 April 2018).

Harvard Health Publishing. (2012). '*Delusional Disorder? What is it?*' /www.health.harvard.edu/search?q=Delusional+Disorder (accessed 31 July 2019).

Insel T (2013). *Transforming diagnosis*. [Blog.] National Institute of Mental Health; 29 April.www.nimh.nih.gov/about/directors/thomas-insel/blog/2013/transforming-diagnosis.shtml (accessed 12 June 2019).

Kiran C, Chaudhury S (2009). Understanding delusions. *Industrial Psychiatry Journal 18*(1): 3–18. www.ncbi.nlm.nih.gov/pmc/articles/PMC3016695/ (accessed 17 April 2018).

Lynch T (2011). *Selfhood: a key to the recovery of emotional and mental wellbeing, and the prevention of mental health problems*. Limerick: Mental Health Publishing.

National Health Service (undated). *Post-traumatic stress disorder*. [Online]. www.nhs.uk/conditions/post-traumatic-stress-disorder-ptsd/causes/ (accessed 18 April 2018).

National Institute of Mental Health (undated-a). *Bipolar disorder*. www.nimh.nih.gov/health/publications/bipolar-disorder/index.shtml (accessed 18 April 2018).

National Institute of Mental Health (undated-b). *Glossary*. www.nimh.nih.gov/health/topics/schizophrenia/raise/glossary.shtml (accessed 17 April 2018).

Rosenberg R (2013). Abnormal is the new normal: why will half of the US population have a diagnosable mental disorder? *Slate*; 12 April. www.slate.com/articles/health_and_science/medical_examiner/2013/04/diagnostic_and_statistical_manual_fifth_edition_why_will_half_the_u_s_population.html (accessed 12 April 2018).

Royal College of Psychiatrists (undated). *Psychosis: information for young people*. www.rcpsych.ac.uk/healthadvice/parentsandyoungpeople/youngpeople/psychosis.aspx (accessed 17 April 2018).

Satir V (1988). *The New Peoplemaking*. Palo Alto, CA: Science and Behavior Books.

Shah N (2015). Self-empowerment. *Huffpost*, 24 June. www.huffingtonpost.com/nipa-shah/self-empowerment_1_b_7647728.html (accessed 16 April 2018).

Silverstone P, Salsali M (2003). Low self-esteem and psychiatric patients: Part I – The relationship between low self-esteem and psychiatric diagnosis. *Annals of General Hospital Psychiatry 2*(2). www.ncbi.nlm.nih.gov/pmc/articles/PMC151271/ (accessed 16 April 2018).

van der Kolk B (2015). *Psychiatry must stop ignoring trauma*. YouTube; 2 February. www.youtube.com/watch?v=HR22lvBo1rQ (accessed 18 April 2018).

World Health Organization (2018). *International Classification of Diseases* (11th revision). Geneva: WHO.

13 | Towards a trauma-informed approach with people who have experienced sexual violence

Lisa Thompson and Becky Willetts

This chapter aims to explain why an understanding of trauma is important when supporting people affected by sexual violence and abuse, and how to implement such an approach in organisations and services. The Rape and Sexual Violence Project (RSVP) is a Birmingham-based charity, covering Solihull too.

At RSVP we offer practical and emotional support to people of any gender affected by sexual violence and abuse. We aim to respond to the children, families and adults in a way that recognises experience and focuses on the individual. As such, our services are grounded in a social trauma model developed by our chairperson, Sally Plumb, from 1992 onwards. Our services and responses aim to validate people's experiences and honour the ways they have tried, and may still be trying, to cope/survive, while also increasing their resilience, coping strategies and wellbeing. A significant part of our work includes recognising and sometimes naming power imbalances. This process alone can be experienced as empowering and can help people to find their own narrative and understanding of their experiences of trauma and how it has affected them.

> RSVP walk with you through the pain. (Client comment)

We believe in the need for society to undergo a fundamental shift in the way we respond to, understand and support sexually abused and exploited children, young people and adults. We need to move away from traditional deficit models (such as the medical model) that explain responses to traumatic experiences as 'disordered', 'mad' or 'bad'.

What do we mean by 'the medical model'?

When discussing the 'medical model' here, we are referring to a construction of health that focuses on deficit, on what is 'wrong' with a person and what needs to be fixed, usually with medication. In relation to physical illness and infection and the need for medicine such as antibiotics to fight them, the medical model or approach can be really helpful. However, in relation to the ways in which people express how they are feeling, and when we enter the realms of mental health, the science becomes less scientific, effective and potentially helpful. We can do biological tests for physical illnesses that will show us what exactly is wrong and what exactly is required to make this better. There are no biological tests for feeling sad, overwhelmed or angry. We have self-reporting measures, but even these are laden with values, judgement and the potential for interpretation by the self or others. This presents significant difficulty when diagnosing and recognising issues to do with mental wellbeing. When someone has experienced sexual trauma, this medical model becomes even more problematic.

Why doesn't it work?

Imagine you are one of the 90% or more of sexually abused or exploited children whose abuser is someone known to them (Radford et al, 2011) – a parent, grandparent, sibling, peer, teacher, religious leader, neighbour etc.

Imagine the likely effects of the trauma and harm of sexual abuse and exploitation, the manipulation of attachments, the misuse of power and control and the dynamics of grooming:

- You may be uncertain about who to trust so you sometimes push people away or you are over-trusting. When relationships that should have been safe, loving and supportive have been unsafe, harmful and abusive, it leaves you confused.
- Your self-confidence may be undermined; you may doubt the validity of your experiences; you may feel responsible for your abuser's behaviours; you may mistrust yourself, others and the wider world.
- You may feel deep shame, believe there is something inherently wrong with you, that you were to blame for the abuse and you are the guilty one, which serves to further attack and erode your self-esteem, worth and confidence.
- Delays, ruptures and halted stages at key points in your development may affect your ability to build resilience, develop safe coping strategies and have good emotional and physical health and wellbeing, not just in childhood but throughout your adult life.
- You may have lifelong difficulties in making safe, secure and supportive attachments in relationships.

Imagine that, in order to seek the help, understanding and support you need, you go/are taken to see your doctor, who prescribes you antidepressants, anti-anxiety medication, stimulants, mood stabilisers and/or antipsychotics. You end up with the message that you, not your abuser(s), are the 'mad', 'bad', 'dangerous', 'ill', 'dysfunctional' or 'disordered' one.

And imagine that this is the best-case scenario. Imagine how it might feel if you were not believed, if you were told that you have made this up, that it's a side effect of your distress, not the cause of it.

Sadly, these are not imaginary situations; they are, rather, the stark reality for many sexually abused and exploited children and young people, and adults too. This is the reality of the medical model. This is the reality of the current society we live in. This is the reality of the often limiting, stigmatising and blaming ways in which we support sexually abused and exploited children, young people and adults, further exacerbating their trauma, distressing experiences and poor emotional wellbeing.

What can we do instead?

When we show professional and personal curiosity in people's experiences and the impact these have had on how they are currently coping, we begin to ask different questions and, hopefully, different answers then follow. A trauma-informed approach is about exploring the impact of people's experiences in order to formulate an understanding of this together, and then addressing any difficulties identified by the person experiencing them. Psychologist and child-trauma specialist Karen Treisman (2018) describes being trauma-informed as:

> … much more than just a 'simple' word or term. It is multi-layered and a whole system approach. It should apply to every sphere of an organisation and be fully embedded into the different levels of a system. This includes integrating trauma-related aspects, knowledge and concepts into things such as training, recruitment, induction, policies, procedures, mission statements, language used, having experts of experience, the environment, team meetings, supervision, reflective practice, leadership style, and so much more!

At RSVP, we use training, resources and communications with children, young people, families, adults and the people supporting them to:

- encourage people to drop the 'disordered' way that they understand and view emotional distress after sexual trauma
- advocate the need for a more affirming, validating and empowering model that emphasises a person's functional, resilient, healthy, understandable, survival responses

- invite people to challenge the overused paradigm that 'mental illness is like any other medical illness', which implies mental distress has a largely biological and genetic base rather than being caused by trauma, adversity and other social and environmental causes

- share how the brain processes traumatic experiences to illustrate how these overwhelming, disempowering, adverse and majorly distressing experiences contribute to people's emotional distress and poor wellbeing, rather than resulting from a 'broken brain', a 'chemical imbalance', or some biological or genetic cause

- show how medical-model responses can exacerbate the belief that there is something wrong with the sexually traumatised and emotionally distressed person, magnifying their feelings of shame, blame, low self-worth, despair and hopelessness

- emphasise that, since abuse happens within relationships, the healing of the harm caused by abuse also needs to happen within a co-created, compassionate, non-abusive, equal, empathic, understanding, warm and supportive relationship with safe boundaries.

Despite the initial overwhelm of considering all the ways in which we can ensure we are delivering trauma-informed services, the real message we think Treisman is trying to convey is that trauma-informed is more than a buzz word/phrase and more than a day's training offered to some staff; it's a whole-organisation approach that will require input, support and change at all levels.

At RSVP we aim to acknowledge the role that trauma and adversity play in the development, onset and enduring nature of emotional distress (eg. feelings that are commonly diagnosed as 'depression' or 'anxiety', suicide attempts etc), especially in childhood, but in adulthood too. Alongside this, we also think it's really important to recognise the impact of childhood trauma and adversity in the development, onset and enduring nature of physical ill health (eg. non-medically explained seizures and chronic pain, migraines etc). The work of the Adverse Childhood Experiences (ACEs) study, 1995–1997 (Felitti et al, 1998) seems to have prompted a growing awareness of this, although corresponding changes in mainstream, statutory mental health and other health systems, services and institutions are non-existent or extremely slow. Access to benefits, services and support are still formulated around medical, 'broken- brain' and 'mental illness' models.

What's the relevance to sexual violence?

In May 2018, Jessica Eaton wrote a blog that focused on the increase of sexually violent language in popular music of most genres (including rap, R&B and more). Eaton also referred to the work of Julia Long (2012) and Gail Dines (2018) on the abundance of easily accessible pornography that not only includes but also seems to glorify sexual violence and abuse. With pornography being accessed at an alarming rate online by such a huge number of people from all walks of life, these worrying trends are becoming normalised, at best, and at worst are influencing a dark and disturbing way of thinking about sex. We are aware of children as young as 13 starting questions with phrases such as, 'When you're raping a girl…' during sex education sessions. Young people's confusion about consent and when it is given and rescinded is expressed in so many forums, from school to the workplace. With sexually violent language commonly used in popular music (for instance, 'beating up' and 'ruining' female genitalia are commonly used phrases), it is to be expected that it will filter into social norms. Music is enjoyed by children, young adults and adults alike, and so language like this becomes how we describe sex, think about sex and potentially have sex.

And? How is this relevant? Why is this relevant? Because we live in a society that is misogynistic and paternalistic and that seeks to place responsibility for sexual violence and abuse on its victims rather than on those who perpetrate the harm. What does it say about our society that anti-rape underwear is available to purchase online? Look at the media reports of rape where the behaviour (drinking/drugs) or clothing of the victim are mentioned. Look at the comments from 'Joe Public', posted online beneath articles where 'actual rape' is condemned, but the behaviour of the 15-year-old girl is described as 'provocative' (that crucial, distancing word loved by the middle classes); where responsibility for reporting the sexual abuse or assault abuse is placed on children who are usually, at best, at risk and at worst already experiencing harm.

Dines (2018) notes:

> A cultural context for understanding why men sexually abuse women, at the levels they do, ironically provides us with hope, because what has been socially constructed can always be socially deconstructed.

Towards a trauma-informed service

At RSVP we are continually working towards becoming a trauma-informed service. We validate experiences (traumatic experiences and memories) rather than focusing on what is 'wrong' with them ('symptoms'), as advocated by traditional approaches.

When seeking to help people understand the ways in which they might respond to threat and fear, we find it can be useful to explain and explore:

- how and where the brain processes trauma (in the amygdala)
- why the brain doesn't respond as people often expect and what the possible psychological impact of this is

- the five defence responses – friend, fight, flight (active) and freeze and flop (passive)
- how services can safely support sexually abused people (especially through disclosure) to avoid further re-traumatisation
- the psychological purpose of guilt, blame and shame
- the potential impact of working with sexual trauma, including secondary and vicarious trauma and the need for self-care
- attachment patterns, and how and why trauma bonds develop and their purpose
- dissociation, dissociative distress and the continuum of dissociation.

As an organisation, we recognise the value of building trust with distressed people, both therapeutically during direct work and in our approach and response at all levels. This means we explain our services and the layout of our organisation fully, so people can see the whole 'menu' of support and information available. We also ensure that we are clear about people's rights and responsibilities when they are in contact with us, to encourage safe relationships that are active rather than passive and involve people in making decisions about the support available to them. We are also working towards co-creation of resources (funds permitting).

We think the concepts behind 'psychological formulation' can be really useful, and that it fits well within a trauma-informed approach as an alternative to medical diagnosis (although we worry that it has become a 'buzz word' and is used as a way to continue diagnosing by a less clinical name). We advise that practitioners using psychological formulation:

- summarise the problems people identify for themselves
- suggest how these problems and difficulties might inter-relate by drawing on psychological theories and principles
- work out, with the distressed person, the best interventions and support strategies for them, based on the psychological processes and principles already identified
- remain flexible, value reflection and revision and be willing to reformulate their understanding of and responses to a person's distress and problems in the light of new information.

We seek to avoid use of medicalised language in our work. This means we do not use terms such as 'treatment', 'patient', 'mad', 'disorder', 'illness', 'broken brain', and any references to 'chemical disorders' or 'imbalances'. We also try to challenge each other within the team, to check out where language comes from, where its roots are and the true meaning of what we are saying.

As an organisation that is working towards implementing a trauma-informed approach, we think it is important that consideration is given to how the support and resources we offer and how we offer them may affect and potentially trigger people's distressing and traumatic experiences. When supporting people who have been subjected to sexual abuse, violence and exploitation, services need to pay particular attention to power dynamics, consent, control, choice, equality and the expertise of people with lived experience. People should be provided with information so they can make their own, informed decisions; services should promote assertiveness (rather than passivity), and organisations should be alert to the risk of vicarious trauma.

It is also important that we acknowledge the sometimes traumatising effects of medical and psychiatric interventions, which can further exacerbate learned helplessness, lack of control, despair, hopelessness and stigma, while simultaneously failing to address the root cause of a person's distress. Once a 'mental illness' has been recognised and 'diagnosed', conventional medical approaches and interventions are usually applied to 'treat' it; to provide sedation, suppressing a person's feelings and potentially their behaviour, without ever trying to understand the context in which 'symptoms' arose in the first place.

It is vital to acknowledge that the behaviours, mood changes and feelings of people who have been sexually abused and exploited do not mean that they are 'mentally ill'. Instead we can reframe this, noting that they may be feeling overwhelming emotional and/or physical distress and that their responses are normal and understandable reactions, strategies and adaptations to the trauma they have been subjected to. While trauma-informed support does not automatically exclude medication, our emphasis is on providing non-medical choices and alternatives that encourage people to use their voices, express not suppress their distress and validate what they did to survive.

It is also important for trauma-informed organisations to consider a wide variety of ways in which sexually traumatised children, young people and adults might want to express their experiences and receive support. It's important that support doesn't just revolve around talking. This can be inappropriate where the abuse has occurred before language developed, difficult because trauma is processed by the more primitive part rather than the logical part of the brain, or simply too distressing for someone to put the horror of their experiences into words. This is where creative interventions such as running, animal-assisted support, art, singing, yoga etc (which have all been offered regularly at RSVP) can be helpful and should be offered. Bessel van der Kolk's research (2014) shows clearly that trauma is embodied; that we hold our experiences within our bodies.

Essentially our practice is rooted in hope and a belief that every sexually abused child, young person and adult has the ability to build on their strengths and assets, grow after trauma and achieve positive outcomes and change, even after early, sadistic, sustained, organised and ritualistic sexual abuse or exploitation.

This is in direct opposition to the medical model messages of the 'lifetime of illness' and 'managing of symptoms' and can be achieved if:

- a person's traumatic experiences are validated
- a person is supported to frame and understand their reactions as healthy, functioning, survival adaptions and responses to trauma
- a person is supported to make sense and meaning of and see the links between what is happening to them now and how it relates to their past.

Through our work, RSVP has and will continue to create training, awareness and resources so that there are more responses, services, organisations, structures and systems where sexually abused children, young people and adults feel validated, heard and believed and where their coping strategies, strengths and assets are honoured, understood and valued not labelled as 'mad', 'bad' and 'ill'.

References

Dines G (2018). Choking women is all the rage. It's branded as fun, sexy 'breath play'. [Blog.] *The Guardian*; 13 May. www.theguardian.com/commentisfree/2018/may/13/choking-women-me-too-breath-play (accessed 5 September 2018).

Eaton J (2018). 'Beat the pussy up' – the way we talk about sex with women. [Blog.] *VictimFocus*; May. www.victimfocus.org.uk/blog (accessed 29 July 2019).

Felitti VJ, Anda RF, Nordenberg D, Williamson DF, Spitz AM, Edwards V, Koss MP, Marks JS (1998). Relationship of childhood abuse and household dysfunction to many of the leading causes of death in adults: the Adverse Childhood Experiences (ACE) study. *American Journal of Preventive Medicine* 14(4): 245–258.

Long J (2012). *Anti-Porn: the resurgence of anti-pornography feminism*. London: Zed Books.

Radford L, Corral S, Bradley C, Fisher H, Bassett C, Howat N, Collishaw S (2011). *Child Abuse and Neglect in the UK Today*. London: NSPCC.

Treisman K (2018). Untitled tweet; 2 March. https://twitter.com/dr_treisman/status/9695597 49325881345?lang=en (accessed 1 August 2019).

van Der Kolk B (2014). *The Body Keeps the Score: mind, brain and body in the transformation of trauma*. New York, NY: Viking.

14 | Disability, depression and the language of disorder

Chris Coombs

I've attempted suicide twice, had thoughts of it many more times, watched my educational career break into tiny pieces, felt at a complete loss as to what to do with my life, been in a couple of car accidents, had a painkiller tube leak after surgery, been threatened with violence. While you'd think that all of these things are frightening, and you'd be right with some of them, any fears pale in comparison to the moment in December 2007 when my mother said, 'I'm taking you to the doctor, I think you have depression.'

That was the moment I knew my life was over. I was a failure, screw-up, dysfunctional, inadequate, a pathetic waste of skin that needed to die. But I was not crazy. I was not a head-case. And here I was in a waiting room, everyone was looking at me, and I was 15 minutes from imprisonment and being put away. As I've become increasingly involved over the years in the conversation about mental health, it can sometimes be difficult to identify with people who still hold in their heads the almighty stigma that exists around these experiences. I'm somewhat inoculated against this because that memory of utter fear of what was going to happen to me when the GP got their hands on me is still very fresh, even now. That crushing feeling of *knowing* with absolute certainty that I was disordered and 'wrong' is something I'll never forget.

Fortunately, a number of things ensured that didn't play out. First, I had a supportive GP who, despite being no mental health expert, did not have the same panicked reaction I did, calmly prescribed antidepressants and put me in line to get some kind of therapy urgently (this was 10 years ago – such things were possible then…). Second, I had a supportive family that wasn't going to cast me aside and onto the scrapheap where I knew I belonged. Third, that family is white, middle class and financially secure – never underestimate those factors, readers; without that extra backing and security at home, I could very easily have gone into a psychiatric ward. My mental health experience of 'the system' is somewhat atypical because of that background. Mental ill health can indeed happen to anyone, it truly knows equality, but certain treatment avenues are more equal than others.

And so I walked away from that appointment with a prescription, a second appointment, some paperwork and a label. 'Depression'.

And, as much as I didn't want that label, it granted solace. It granted some relief. It proved that this was not my fault. That what I had was some dodgy brain chemistry, allied with a lot of stress, and that, if both those things could be sorted, normalcy would once again emerge. It was an explanation, and in that time when I was completely and utterly lost, it was important, precious and much needed. From that moment I was split. I knew there was a part of me, the depressive part, that would fight help all the way; that would creep in if I was not vigilant and active and, like a large spider, lurk in a dark corner, to be discovered with shock and fear. But that was still kind of OK. Because in our culture we talk so much about self-improvement, about resilience, about character traits – as if a personality were something that could be tinkered with just enough to get the most desirable results and a much-sought-after 'balance' (a particularly in-vogue phrase even now that I urge you to view with suspicion).

And so, with that in the background, 'depression' and I waged war. Sometimes I won, sometimes it won. There was The Battle of Sertraline (inconclusive), The Great Choral Campaigns of 2010, 2012 and 2013 – periods when singing and performing served as a survival strategy – (I won), The Employment Front (depression won – and handily) – all titanic struggles, but the two sides remained evenly matched. In 2014, a truce was called, the Citalopram Protocol was implemented, to the annoyance of both sides, and the treaty was signed. All was well for about eight months, and then 'depression' launched a surprise attack that almost knocked me out of the war. Having been under siege for most of 2015, I sallied forth with a new round of therapy that lasted for eight months. And with that added companion, I had a chance to actually look at my enemy.

What I found was startling.

Mental health diagnosis gives us a kind of mechanistic answer to the question 'how?' How did I end up the way I am? And, with its focus on brain chemistry, physical health and the relationship between the two, it gives us the idea that, again, if some kind of equilibrium is achieved, then the rest will fall into place. In this image of mental experience, it's as if the body is a well-oiled machine with a very literal screw loose. Fix that screw and the rest will take care of itself. Except the rest wasn't taking care of itself. Moreover, none of this bore any relevance to what I was talking to my therapist about. We're at a point where we're overflowing with good mental health 'tips', but ask someone who's struggling why it is that they are where they are, and rarely do they answer, 'My nutrition is completely out of whack' or 'I'm just not getting the right work-life balance' or 'I'm just not taking enough time for me'. These things are useful – but often it's fiddling at the edges of a problem. We talk about 'mental illnesses' as just that – 'illnesses' – because it's easier to deal with these things through the lens of health. Cancer can happen to anyone, illnesses can strike anyone, 'mental ill health' can strike anyone. It is a random thing, we're told, borne out of a genetic lottery. But rare is the client who says to a therapist, 'Yeah, it's the dodgy genes that are the problem.' Clients actually talk about everything else – their emotions, feelings, life circumstances, oppressive experiences, traumas, grief, loss and a whole host of other things.

At the back end of 2015, as I started out on a new leg of my therapy journey, I looked at 'depression'. Where did it come from? What was it about? Had I been honest to say it was simply a part of me? Yes and no…

It was everywhere, but it was borne out of much more than simple biology. Out of academic expectations not met, self-imposed rules and introjections, never *really* addressing some of the effects of being suicidal. A lack of direction, a lack of meaning, a lack of relationship and, quietly in the background, a creeping realisation that all was not well with my view of my own body and disability and my actually diagnosable condition of cerebral palsy and the idea that my body was older than I felt. There was so much more to it even than all that, and the complex interplay is something I could never hope to translate fully, but all this led to a simple realisation. 'Depression' wasn't so much about my body and brain mechanics, but about *what happened to me*.

Part of the reason I think so many people cling to diagnostic labels is that they think their stories are unworthy of their feelings and emotions. A label takes that out of their hands. Labels mean that we don't have to question whether someone's mental health struggles are somehow legitimate or acceptable. We don't have to see if they tick enough boxes to be helped or treated. The label covers for that.

But, if we are any kind of caring society, should we even have to ask if someone's experiences and responses are somehow *fair*? The worst thing that happens to a person is the worst thing that happened to them. Who are we to say whether or not that qualifies for a label and a diagnosis? What experiences are toxic enough to 'need' treating, and which ones are acceptable? Who are we to say when a grief or low mood is invalid because it has passed the sell-by date and is now a pathology? This shit is too damn personal for that. And because that is entirely personal, I now find the label of 'depression' cumbersome and unwieldy. I've not come to that overnight – it is a long journey that is not finished. But I have come to realise that, based on who I am, my reactions to everything were understandable and made logical sense. Those responses to trauma are mine and mine alone. My emotions and feelings and subsequent actions were not a result of being somehow 'disordered', but natural human reactions that had no need to be pathologised or placed in the box marked 'wrong'.

I experience that same sense of disjunction between how I feel and the labels I am expected to use to describe my feelings when it comes to my disability. Due to many medical interventions over the years, my body has not always felt like it belonged to me.

Disabled friends and acquaintances from as far back as my school days have expressed similar sentiments – that they've felt objectified and dissociated when being observed, manhandled or manipulated in medical settings. I use the word *dissociated* here, to make things easier to follow and understand, but I'm not entirely happy with it. I've written in the past about feeling grotesque in my disabled body, and disgusted and unhappy with it; some friends have identified similar feelings and experiences, describing themselves as *dysmorphic.* That is their right, but again this is a word that I don't feel entirely happy using. And the major reason for my discomfort with both of these terms is that both are rooted in that language of disorder.

'Dysmorphia' and 'dissociation', like 'anxiety' and 'depression', are terms that are easy enough for the average member of the public to grasp within a few minutes' conversation. They can help to explain complex human experiences. As much as we can overuse them, labels can perform a useful shorthand role. The problem is that they also bring those connotations of 'mental illness', 'disorder' and wrongness, if they aren't explored in depth and with considerable nuance. Because of our cultural heritage of framing mental distress as 'illness', there is an automatic bias that any kind of mental stormy weather is a 'disorder'. I've discovered this again recently, as I've been scouring the internet for resources, articles and stories about disabled people who 'dissociate' in the same or similar ways that I do, or have felt at some point that strange sense of body 'dysmorphia' (interestingly, it's very hard to find Google results for body *dysphoria*, though in my case that's what I feel is more apt), where they have felt that their bodies were not entirely theirs and were repulsed by certain aspects of them. In searching for shared experiences, it has struck me over and over again that the entire narrative is rooted in medical 'disorder'. Simply typing 'body dysmorphia' into Google will yield reams of results all about 'body dysmorphic disorder (BDD)' – you'll notice, I didn't search for the 'disorder' part of that story. Similarly, if you type '*dissociation from body*' into the same search engine, the list of immediate results are *all* about 'dissociative disorders'. Again – the 'disorders' bit was not in my search term.

Because I've been lucky enough to have conversations with and move in adjacent circles to many people who are critical of this type of framework, I have come away frustrated more than anything else. If I'd been unfamiliar with alternative views, I might well have reached a conclusion that I had yet another mental health diagnosis of 'BDD' or 'DD' to add to a growing list of acronyms. And I feel very lucky to not have to go down that pathway, because it means that I can keep exploring all of the avenues of my experience in my journey towards making meaning. If I had taken the view that the acronyms were the key point, then everything else would have had to be framed to fit alongside them. And that would be a shame, because the more I think about these things, the dissociation and body dysphoria that I sometimes experience, the anxiety, the depressive episodes, I don't think of them as medical issues. I see them more and more as human responses to things that have happened to me and around me.

Take dissociation for instance. In my current view, I see it as a reaction. I dissociate in medical settings because I don't feel I am of much importance in the room. My *body* is but, particularly when I was growing up, my thoughts, feelings and opinions on what was happening to me, or being done to me, were almost never sought. That's not a criticism in itself, merely a statement of fact. And so, in that environment, I shut down, because I felt that, while my body was the focus, it was a deeply depersonalising process. I switch off because it's easier to go somewhere else than to deal with the complex paradox of wanting to be present and involved with the process now as an adult but feeling awful discomfort in doing so. My brain goes elsewhere because being manhandled, even for positive purposes, can sometimes feel invasive. I go blank because I've experienced walking up and down rooms countless times under observation from people who in their own way wanted to *fix* what was *wrong* with my walking, and in those circumstances it's easier to mentally go elsewhere than engage with that sense of feeling *otherness* and *wrongness*. Is this disordered on my part? I don't feel so. It feels like a bunch of coping strategies that I've only recently noticed, some of which I will doubtless keep and some of which I will likely change, but 'disordering' my responses serves nothing except a narrative that accepts a cultural status quo.

So, what about my sporadic sense of body 'dysphoria'? Surely the language of disorder fits when an individual feels out of place with or uncomfortable in their own skin? I beg to differ. First, my body is fundamentally different to the vast majority of people's in that it does not do things such as run or stand still comfortably without a huge amount of focus, concentration, extra co-ordination or, in the case of running, expenditure of energy. While I have come to a place where I can for the most part get by and lead a relatively normal life, I am aware every waking moment that I am different from most other people. The societal norm of bodies does not match up with mine, and existing in a world that looks at things through an abled lens has led to me internalising vast amounts of ableism throughout my upbringing. This was largely not something I was aware of until the latter stages of 2017, but nevertheless internalised ableism has played a huge factor in some of the negative ways that I have thought about my own physicality. Alongside this has been an actually legitimate emotional cocktail comprised mostly of grief, rage and a sense of loss for the limitations that cerebral palsy has left me with. These are merely the main factors in my constantly changing relationship to my own body, but I'm sure you can see that it's a multi-faceted and deeply tangled web of feelings, emotions, social, medical and political factors. With this amount of background noise, I now consider that the sporadic periods where I feel a great deal of uncertainty and lack of identity with my physical body are a fair-enough response. The medical terms of diagnosis – 'dysmorphic disorder' chief among them – do nothing for an explanation that makes sense to me, and merely betray a paucity of language and a lack of understanding within much of the mental health world.

Because calling someone 'disordered' is nothing more than putting blame for their experiences on their shoulders.

And one of the things that's most galling about the dominant narrative of diagnosis is that it leaves no room in the discussion for alternative views of human pain, suffering and distress – it exists often in the realms of pure dogma. And while this leaves a multitude of problems, I'd like to use this space to highlight one in particular. There is no roadmap for people who are discovering and exploring aspects of their experience for the first time to talk about things in terms other than the diagnostic. I would desperately love to talk to other disabled people about how we relate to our own bodies, how they see things like autonomy, their sense of self, ownership of their bodies, do they feel negative or positive about them, where is the line between justifiable anger and internalised ableism, has their view changed as they've aged and transitioned between child and adult services and environments, how does this relate to sexuality, how does it relate to self-image and self-esteem… And those are just the questions that immediately occur to me!

But every time I write about my own journey, I feel like I am skydiving, jumping out of a plane with a slightly worn-looking parachute. It may well be fine, but it feels like an enormous risk with each jump, because I often don't know if others feel remotely like me and I have to wait until after the jump for confirmation, or otherwise. Before every jump, the only voices and stories I hear are those rooted in 'disorder' and 'mental illness'. And I know that this does not fit me. I'm learning on the job how to talk about my sense of self. We need to reclaim the language surrounding this. If we don't, then we risk never fully exploring our most fundamental experiences and questions. The lens of disorder can only take us so far. When it has ceased to be useful, we should look elsewhere.

15 | Finding my tribe: a survivor's story

Sue Irwin

The feeling of not belonging is a sign you are supposed to be somewhere else,
doing something different.
Let it push you.
Let it shove you.
Let it force you onto a new path.
(Anonymous)

This chapter represents my reflections after attending five A Disorder for Everyone! (AD4E)[1] events and from my membership of the Facebook group 'Drop the Disorder!'[2] My perspective comes from my experiences not only as a survivor of childhood abuse and the mental health system, but also as a woman, a mother, a sister and many other life situations in which I have found myself.

It's true to say that I've procrastinated about writing this piece – gathering together my thoughts, assembling a writing space and an environment that feels comfortable and inspiring, even waiting for the sun to appear from behind the clouds. I've sat in front of my computer for many hours wondering where I should begin. At the beginning would be the obvious place, but where is that? Is it when I first came across the name 'Jo Watson' and, on reading her profile, felt her infectious passion rising up inside me too? Is it when I first came into contact with mental health professionals 21 years ago? Is it the day I came into this world

---

1. www.adisorder4everyone.com (accessed 29 June 2019)

2. www.adisorder4everyone.com/new-facebook-group (accessed 29 June 2019)

as an innocent baby or, indeed, when time itself began? I'm not sure, but as so often happens these days, I have chosen to start at a place of safety.

Throughout my life I had often felt the odd one out, that I was somehow different to those around me – the 'ugly duckling' of my family and the community in which I lived. Although a shy, quiet and introverted child, whose soul had been bruised and battered, there lay buried somewhere deep within me a spirit that I have come to call the warrior Sue, and she has proved vital for my survival throughout my life. I often spent my time on the periphery of peer groups, never feeling accepted by or part of the clan and rarely participating or feeling comfortable in the social activities that came with growing up in the 1960s and 70s.

My feelings of alienation continued as this somewhat solitary childhood existence progressed into adolescence and then on into adulthood, when that alienation would be deepened even further by 18 years of treatment under mainstream mental health services.

It was with a refreshing sense of vitality and relief, then, that one late spring morning in May 2016, while casually searching the internet for inspiration and understanding of my experiences, I happened to stumble across a page advertising an event that seemed to be speaking my language and whispering to my soul. As I scrolled through the booking process, I wondered if this could be the tribe I had unconsciously been searching for since early childhood. Somebody called Jo Watson was organising a conference not far from my home and, having read the outline of the day, I certainly wasn't going to miss this one. I booked a place and paid for my ticket in an instant. 'A Disorder for Everyone! – Exploring the Culture of Psychiatric Diagnoses' was coming to a town near me.

Living in exile

I had grown up in an ordinary family, the youngest of three siblings, attended ordinary state schools, gained average grades in exams and a degree in European languages. I found employment, married and gave birth to two beautiful and unique daughters. At the age of 35, I became pregnant with my third child (a son) and to the outside world and to me my life appeared straightforward.

Despite my feelings of alienation, I excelled in fitting in and conforming to the norms of the world in which I lived, and I survived this existence by looking outside of myself, not daring to delve into what lay beneath my skin, denying what had happened to me and simply getting on with life. But there lay a secret within me, a secret from childhood that was buried so deeply inside my subconscious that it rarely surfaced. I was made to believe that the consequences of sharing this secret would be devastating, that no one would believe me and I would be seen as wicked and crazy for telling such stories. So, whenever questions were asked of me about my early years and I contemplated sharing this secret, a sense of terror and shame would often engulf me, so much so that I remained silent – or, rather,

I was silenced. This secret was to lie dormant but festering within me until the birth of my son.

Shortly after his birth, and with three young children to care for, I found myself unable to manage the unfamiliar confusion and distress I was experiencing. Believing that I could trust in the expertise of professionals, I willingly turned to my GP and then to statutory mental health services for help. I was immediately given the first of many psychiatric diagnoses, together with a prescription for antidepressants to treat my 'symptoms', and so began a journey that was to last 17 long and at times desperate years.

By the time my son was about to celebrate his 17th birthday, I was one of those infamous revolving-door patients and defined myself simply as a set of numbers from the *Diagnostic and Statistical Manual of Mental Disorders* (American Psychiatric Association, 2013). Locked hospital wards had become my second home; I was dependent on doctors, nurses, cocktails of medication and ECT, and believed that this was the only way to keep alive and existing – any sense of personal agency or responsibility had been extinguished.

Sadly, I had been unable to find an environment that felt safe enough for me to communicate the true cause of my distress. Instead of helping me to explore, make sense of and understand the reasons and causes of my intense distress, the diagnoses and labels I was given simply left me feeling that my very core was being questioned. I felt my experiences of abuse were being ignored and somehow irrelevant; I felt more ashamed and guilty, and I felt I was to blame for responding to trauma in ways that were judged as negative, irrational, inappropriate, destructive and harmful. Yet, from my perspective, I felt I was reacting sanely to an insane situation.

What I didn't realise at the time, however, was that the power imbalances within the mental health system, especially between doctor and patient, mirrored the powerless situation I found myself in as a child, where the misuse of power had posed a very real threat to me.

My responses to that threat manifested in ways such as disconnection both from myself and the world around me, self-harm, suicidal thoughts and attempts, the abuse of alcohol and cannabis, anger and, at the same time, meekness and submissiveness, as well as an intense need to please others. And, rather than those responses being seen as sophisticated coping mechanisms that I was using in order to survive, they were seen as 'symptoms' of an illness, a 'disorder' or a 'syndrome', 'symptoms' to be got rid of with pills and electricity by a mental health system that seemed intent on medicalising my distress. And so, after almost two decades of being caught in the mental health system, the abuser's words seemed to have come true – I believed and felt that not only was I 'mad', but I was also 'bad'.

My feelings of alienation had now grown into a poisonous, overwhelming and almost unbearable sense of loneliness. This, coupled with a toxic sense of self-loathing, self-disgust, self-invested anger, hopelessness and despair, seemed to have successfully broken my spirit. I believed the time had come for me to put a permanent end to this misery and I came up with a solid plan to take my own life. I decided on the method I would use and chose my parents' graveside as a comforting place to spend my final moments. I did my best to write a meaningful letter to each of my children in an effort to explain my actions. I organised my finances so that my family would not have to worry about the cost of funeral expenses, and I went to a solicitor to organise a will. But the warrior in me – essentially, the essence of me – would not allow me to carry out my plan. Having been admitted to an acute hospital ward once again, it was decided that I should come off, overnight, the cocktail of psychiatric medications I had been taking for 17 years, and my world was turned upside down. While this rather brutal decision was made for me and I had no choice in the matter, it proved to be a momentous turning point in my life.

Coming out of exile

'A journey of a thousand miles begins with a single step.' So the *Tao Te Ching* tells us. As I look back on my life so far, I see that there have been points in time that I would describe as 'defining moments' – moments that would guide me down a path of my own choosing, although sometimes it felt as if I had no choice. Some of those paths proved helpful and purposeful, but, sadly, some turned out not to have been so positive. I'm happy to admit that, just like anyone else, I've made many mistakes along the way, although I like to think that I have learnt from some of them. I've also encountered an array of colourful and diverse characters who I can honestly say have made a positive difference to my life.

But, without hesitation, I can say that the most defining moment of my life to date was the moment when I was taken off all psychiatric medication. There is no doubt in my mind that, had this life-changing event not happened, I would no longer be alive today to tell my story – such was the hopelessness I felt. This was the moment, at the age of 53, when I began to take the first tentative and small steps on my painful and challenging journey of healing from the wounds that had been inflicted on me by others – some intentionally and some unintentionally.

The psychiatrist who made the decision to take me off all medication had advised me that I might experience a few weeks of withdrawal symptoms, but as I look back on that time, it's clear to me now that my whole being went into a state of shock. After so many years of adapting to these toxic chemicals, my mind and body were desperately trying to readjust and find their own state of natural equilibrium. Little did I know that it would take more than just a few weeks to heal from this trauma.

As I slowly emerged from this state of shock, I began to realise the enormity of the debilitating and spellbinding effects that years of medication had cast upon me and the negative impact that the mental health system as a whole had had on my life. Despite the turmoil and agony of withdrawal, the fog seemed to lift and my thoughts became clearer. After 17 years under the care of mental health professionals, I had become a great deal sicker, both physically and psychologically. I felt I had lost 17 years of my life; I had scant if any memories of the first precious years of my children's lives and of the final years of my parents' lives. How could a system I had turned to for help have harmed me like this?

It just did not make sense to me and, as my questions were met with what felt like a wall of silence, my disbelief turned into rage, my sadness into grief and my confusion into curiosity, determination and passion. I made it my mission to find out how this could have happened in an effort to ensure that others would not have to experience what I had endured. I also realised that the only way forward for me was to take on responsibility for my future, and this felt somewhat overwhelming, as I'd become dependent on services. But, being a warrior, I was determined to prove others wrong and carve out a life that suited me and where I felt able to make my own choices. In order for that to happen, the first step I needed to take was to liberate myself from mainstream mental health services and wave goodbye to the revolving-door patient that was once me.

Discovery

Marcel Proust is credited as saying, 'The only real voyage of discovery… consists not in seeing new landscapes, but in having new eyes' (O'Brien, 1948). This is so true for me. Soon after parting company with the mental health services, I began walking along two distinct pathways. The first was to seek out someone to help me heal from the wounds I had been subjected to, and I very quickly found an experienced trauma therapist in private practice – that therapy still continues. The second was to attend a training course in peer support that would open my eyes to a new way of thinking about this thing called 'mental illness'.

Although it only involved 11 days of training, it was nevertheless incredibly informative, intense and inspiring, and even transformative for me. I discovered that there were many conflicting ideas and perspectives about human distress and our responses to it. I read stories, articles and papers written by survivors and was signposted to organisations such as Mad in America[3] and the Hearing Voices Network.[4] I learnt about the history of peer support and what 'recovery' might mean, and there were discussions about the language we use.

But, most importantly, I learnt a great deal about me, and I experienced a real sense of personal growth. For the first time in many, many years, I felt curious, my thirst for knowledge rose to an unprecedented level, a sense of hope began to grow within me, and I felt excited!

I went on to gain an accredited qualification in peer support and successfully applied for a job as a peer support worker with my local mental health service,

3. www.madinamerica.com (accessed 29 June 2019)
4. www.hearing-voices.org (accessed 29 June 2019)

working on the acute ward where I had previously been a patient. It was a massively empowering and liberating experience to be working alongside people who had once witnessed me in my darkest moments. But I very quickly began to sense a moral conflict developing inside me and, after 12 months, I resigned from my post, unable to continue working within a system where I felt my values, authenticity and integrity were being compromised.

It was around the time of my resignation that I attended the first AD4E event in Birmingham, and what an experience that proved to be. I had met up with another attendee the previous evening, eager to find out what others felt and what had led them to attend. It also helped that I would then know someone at the event and perhaps find safety in sitting next to them.

As I sat in the audience, surrounded by people who seemed to be thinking the way I had come to think about my own experiences of distress, and listening to speakers who I felt were talking complete sense, I felt an immediate sense of safety. Finally, I thought, these are people who are most definitely speaking my language. A feeling of relief came over me as I realised that I was not alone and that I was not after all an ugly duckling.

I went on to attend four more AD4E events in 2018 and 2019 – Brighton, Birmingham, London and Wolverhampton – I always feel at home. The range of speakers and topics covered would reinforce my feelings that change was needed and that the seeds of that change were already planted and beginning to spread their roots. Each event was unique and, despite the highly emotive themes being discussed and the impact that might have on me as a survivor, I found myself drawn to attend – feeling as if I were with family meant that I felt safe to be me.

Connecting globally – Drop the Disorder!

Shortly before the first AD4E Birmingham event, I was directed to the closed Facebook group, Drop the Disorder!. Having recently signed up to this new way of connecting with people, other than face to face or over the telephone, I felt somewhat nervous at what felt for me to be a rather impersonal way of communicating. But I was surprised by how my sense of belonging improved from joining this group.

The group membership grew rapidly, and it very quickly became a place for me to seek sanctuary and knowledge. From being a suspicious onlooker, I soon became an active observer and, from time to time, I was even able to find the courage to place a post or comment on one of the discussion topics. My trepidation about posting anything about myself or my own opinions initially came from the belief that I was not an expert, but simply a 'mentally ill' patient with little insight and nothing of value to offer in discussions. This feeling soon passed as I read posts and comments from the diverse range of people within the group, who I felt showed incredible passion, compassion and respect for individual experiences, thoughts and opinions. I found the group members open and inclusive.

Many differing theories, viewpoints and perspectives were introduced on a daily basis and, as time went on, I would feel almost compelled to log in each evening – curious and excited to read about the day's topics. I'd compare this feeling to being like a small child in a sweet shop, not knowing which jar of sweets to choose. That feeling was quite foreign to me.

There were times, however, when I found myself reaching for the dictionary in an effort to understand the language being used, and it was sometimes difficult for me to make sense of what was being discussed and/or the theories being introduced. As someone who was and still is working through my own trauma in person-centred therapy, I found the theories somewhat confusing and would sometimes bring to therapy some of the ideas I'd read about in the group. My therapist showed great humility and would always welcome my questions and concerns, commenting that, despite being in practice for many years, she was always grateful and willing to learn new ideas and perspectives from clients.

There were moments too when discussions became heated and certain posts felt too emotive for me. So, to protect myself, I chose to spend less time following and reading through posts, giving myself space to focus on my world closer to home.

Reflections

My overriding feelings about the AD4E and Drop the Disorder! Facebook group are that it has given me a sense of belonging that has been missing for most of my life and this has played an important part in my own healing journey and my experience of post-traumatic growth. I have come into contact with people who have shared their own stories of distress and given me the courage, confidence and inspiration to speak out and find my own voice. I have been given space to share my own story in a safe environment and gone on to tell it in wider settings, in the hope of creating change. I have read about many new and interesting ideas, theories and perspectives, which in turn has helped me to identify, build upon and believe in my own worldview. And I have found other, like-minded human beings who have helped to restore my faith in humanity.

Thanks to these experiences, then, for the foreseeable future, one of my missions is to continue telling my story and to try to plant the seeds of change at a grassroots level. I like to think that I have dropped the 'disordered patient' role and taken on the role of gardener in a team, helping to create a diverse garden full of flourishing flowers.

References

American Psychiatric Association (2013). *The Diagnostic and Statistical Manual of Mental Disorders* (5th ed). Washington, DC: APA.

O'Brien J (ed) (1948). *The Maxims of Marcel Proust*. New York, NY: Columbia University Press (p181).

16 | From chemical imbalance to power imbalance: a manifesto for mental health

Peter Kinderman

In June 2017, the United Nations' Special Rapporteur, Dainius Pūras, a child psychiatrist from Lithuania, presented a report to the UN Human Rights Council setting out 'the core challenges and opportunities for advancing the realization of the right to mental health of everyone'. In it, he argued:

> For decades, mental health services have been governed by a reductionist biomedical paradigm… Mental health policies should address the 'power imbalance' rather than 'chemical imbalance'. (Pūras, 2017)

Making this change will be a challenge. And, if we are to challenge decades of messages from the pharmaceutical industries and professions with vested interests, and to change ideas about mental health in the media and general public that are now well established, we need to have a clear alternative. I am going to attempt this here.

First, though, I want to unpick the rationale for such a momentous reform of an age-old system of abuse and exploitation.

Brains and biology

All our thoughts, behaviours and emotions reflect the biological activity of our brains, but this does not mean that 'mental health problems' need therefore to be regarded as brain diseases. The delivery of mental health services must be based on the premise that our psychological wellbeing depends on the things that happen to us, how we make sense of those events and how we respond to them. The assertion that our distress is best understood as a 'symptom' of diagnosable 'illnesses' is only one perspective, and a rather unhelpful one. Instead of relying on this 'disease model', which assumes that emotional distress is a 'symptom' of biological illness, we need to embrace and implement a compassionate, social and psychological approach to mental health and wellbeing that recognises our essential and shared humanity.

It is a simple fact of life that all our thoughts, behaviours and emotions emanate from the biological activity of our brains. But this does not mean that 'mental health problems' therefore need to be regarded as 'symptoms' of a brain disease. Our brains have evolved to allow us to process information about the world and make sense of our environment. These neurological mechanisms underpin all psychological processes, whether 'depression', 'anxiety', falling in love, writing poetry, or going to war. We should try to understand the involvement of neurotransmitters, of synapses and neurones in human behaviour, not assume that 'mental health problems' are purely the result of biological disorders.

Making sense of the world

We need a functioning brain to make emotional sense of the world, but the ways in which we develop our own framework of understanding is far from biologically determined.

Our mental health reflects our thoughts about ourselves, other people, the world and the future. These 'cognitive schemas' are formed in response to our experiences in life; they are learned, not biologically determined. Of course, how we make sense of the world has consequences for our mood and our behaviour – even our physiological status. But that is true for a whole range of issues, as anyone attending a rock concert, a religious ceremony, a marriage, a court case or an employment tribunal could testify. Our past experiences affect how we experience and interpret things that happen in the present.

Our brains allow us to learn, rather than dictate our behaviours. This learning certainly occurs via biological pathways, but that does not imply that differences between us can be meaningfully reduced to biological differences (Kinderman, 2014).

We don't merely react passively to life events; our response is dependent on our physical substrate – our environment. Learning is core to the human experience, and our learning is abstract, complex and cognitive. We build mental models of the world through our experiences and our relationships and by learning from others, through the conscious and unconscious development of meaning. Events impact on our mental health through their effects on our psychological mechanisms.

One of the supreme accomplishments of the evolution of the human brain is the capacity for abstract thought. We have an enormous capacity for learning.

We humans made the huge evolutionary leap of developing the ability to extract abstract, meaningful representations of the world. And these abstractions have significant implications for our emotions and behaviour, even our subsequent thought processes. We learn to predict the future and understand the rules behind schedules of reinforcement. More than that, we learn to understand problems and solve them, rather than merely act in the hope of reward. We also model our behaviour on that of other people; we learn the rules of social behaviour. What we believe about ourselves, our abilities, strengths and weaknesses, what we hope – or fear – for the future and what we believe about the nature of the world, especially the social world, are all crucial to our mental health. A belief that someone close to us is untrustworthy, or even dangerous, really does matter. Similarly, it absolutely matters if we believe that there is no hope, no future, no point in carrying on living.

What we learn to believe, how we have ended up thinking about the world, how we have learned to make sense of the world, is profoundly important. It has real causal power. If someone believes that their life has no meaning, and that the future is bleak, then there are profound consequences. But these beliefs do not arise as a 'symptom' of an 'illness'. There are reasons why we view the world in the ways we do. And that's why these psychological issues are so fundamentally important.

Labels are for products, not people

The traditional diagnostic system risks pathologising nearly all aspects of our lives, with the inevitable danger that we are 'treated' for normal psychological phenomena as though they were medical illnesses. The risks are greater for children, whose brains are still developing, who are at the start of their learning about life and the world around them.

The criteria for psychiatric diagnoses are not only scientifically perplexing but also deeply worrying, because of their implications for care. It is important to recognise that children and adults occasionally experience very serious problems. Criticism of the diagnostic approach does not mean 'domesticating' people's problems or pretending they don't exist. Quite the opposite. We should acknowledge the deep reality of the difficulties that some adults and children face. But such recognition is undermined if all we do is attempt to fit these problems into a disease model.

We should be worried that, in the US in 2014, more than 80,000 prescriptions were issued for antidepressants for children aged two and younger; that 20,000 prescriptions for antipsychotic medication were made out for the same age group (Schwarz, 2015). In the UK, nearly a million prescriptions for Ritalin and related drugs for 'attention deficit hyperactivity disorder' ('ADHD') were dispensed in 2017 – more than double the number a decade previously (Boffey, 2015). In the US, the numbers are even higher.

Most psychological phenomena lie along continua, from the least to the most serious problems. Generally, scientific analyses of the distribution of psychological problems have failed to find clear distinctions between the supposedly diagnosable 'illnesses'. Most research shares the conclusions of Godfrey Pearlson and Judith Ford (2014), that there is 'no point of symptomatic rarity between schizophrenia, psychotic bipolar disorder, and schizoaffective disorder' and 'the boundaries between clinical entities defined by phenomenology appear to be distributed on a continuum and to lack sharp demarcations'. In plain words, there are no distinct disease entities that can be labelled 'schizophrenia', 'bipolar disorder' or 'schizoaffective disorder' – their identifiable symptoms merge, overlap and flow between these artificial categorisations.

Rejection of the diagnostic approach opens up the prospect of humane and rational approaches to care. It dispels the stigma of 'them' (the mentally diseased) and 'us' (the well ones). Among many other campaigners, the Only Us Campaign challenges the idea of 'them' and 'us' and instead proposes that:

> … there's a continuum, a scale along which we all slide back and forth during our lives, sometimes happy, occasionally depressed or very anxious; mostly well balanced but with moody moments; usually in touch with reality, but at times detached or even psychotic. When we separate ourselves and imagine humanity divided into two different groups, we hurt those labelled as sick, ill, even mad. We allow stigma, prejudice and exclusion to ruin potentially good and creative lives. But we also hurt ourselves, because we stress ourselves out with false smiles and the suppression of our own vulnerabilities. There is no them and us, THERE'S ONLY US.[1]

Real world experiences and social context

Rather than use medical, pathologising language and methods, we can and should use effective, scientific, understandable alternatives. An alternative to psychiatric diagnosis would be simply to list a person's experiences in their own terms. Such a straightforward approach would enable our problems to be recognised (in both senses of the word), understood, validated, explained, and allow us to develop a plan for help.

Moreover, despite being rarely discussed, used or reported either in clinical practice or in the academic literature (Allsopp & Kinderman, 2017), the existing World Health Organization coding system includes descriptive information about adverse life experiences and living environments. In *ICD-11* (World Health Organization, 2018), for example, these quasi-diagnostic codes document such

1. See https://twitter.com/onlyuscampaign (accessed 29 July 2019)

factors as a personal history of sexual abuse (QE82.1) or a history of spouse or partner violence (QE51.1).

This gives us a much more appropriate alternative to the use of quasi-medical psychiatric diagnoses. It is possible, using *ICD-11*, to offer a diagnosis of 'Moderate Personality Disorder' (6D10.1), but I wouldn't recommend it. Not only is it insulting (as it defines a person's personality as 'disordered') and serves to locate fault within the individual, rather than looking at the root causes of the difficulties; it is also unnecessary. It is possible, instead, to record formally one or more adverse or traumatic experiences and subsequent specific mental health difficulties. For example, you can record personal history of sexual abuse (QE82.1), history of spouse or partner violence (QE51.1), and low income (QD51), leading (understandably) to anger (MB24.1), depressed mood (MB24.5), feelings of guilt (MB24.B), and non-suicidal self-injury (MB23.E).

I believe such social determinant and phenomenological codes offer a constructive, radical way forward (Kinderman & Allsopp, 2018). Such an approach would be far more informative and honest, and far less pathologising, than the diagnostic status quo. It would also meet the legitimate requirement for appropriate, internationally recognised data collection and shared language, while avoiding the inadequacies of reliability and validity associated with traditional diagnoses.

A new ethos

The changes I am arguing for do not only draw their support from the radical fringe. In 2012, the World Health Organization maintained that the way that societies globally care for people with mental health problems constitutes a hidden human rights emergency (World Health Organization, 2012). Implementation of the United Nations' Convention on the Rights of Persons with Disabilities (2006) is monitored by a body of independent experts known as special rapporteurs, appointed by the Human Rights Council. Dainius Pūras' report (2017), which I quoted from at the start of this chapter, is based on sound psychological science and is earth-shattering in its honesty. Among its observations, it says:

> For decades, mental health services have been governed by a reductionist biomedical paradigm that has contributed to the exclusion, neglect, coercion and abuse of people with intellectual, cognitive and psychosocial disabilities, persons with autism and those who deviate from prevailing cultural, social and political norms… We have been sold a myth that the best solutions for addressing mental health challenges are medications and other biomedical interventions… Public policies continue to neglect the importance of the preconditions of poor mental health, such as violence, disempowerment, social exclusion and isolation and the breakdown of

communities, systemic socioeconomic disadvantage and harmful conditions at work and in schools… Reductive biomedical approaches to treatment that do not adequately address contexts and relationships can no longer be considered compliant with the right to health.

The report condemns the neglect of 'the preconditions of poor mental health, such as violence, disempowerment, social exclusion and isolation and the breakdown of communities, systemic socioeconomic disadvantage and harmful conditions at work and in schools.' There is, it declares, 'an almost universal commitment to pay for hospitals, beds and medications instead of building a society in which everyone can thrive.' It gives a stern warning about the dangers of encouraging the unrestricted export of a Western, psychiatric, disease-model approach to mental health that promotes technical diagnosis, biological explanations and a reliance on pharmacological interventions. 'An effective tool used to elevate global mental health is the use of alarming statistics to indicate the scale and economic burden of "mental disorders"; it says. Furthermore:

> The current 'burden of disease' approach firmly roots the global mental health crisis within a biomedical model, too narrow to be proactive and responsive in addressing mental health issues at the national and global level. The focus on treating individual conditions inevitably leads to… narrow, ineffective and potentially harmful outcomes… [and] paves the way for further medicalization of global mental health, distracting policymakers from addressing the main risk and protective factors affecting mental health for everyone… The scaling-up of care must not involve the scaling-up of inappropriate care.

Drawing on a range of examples and resources, including the British Psychological Society's report *Understanding Psychosis and Schizophrenia* (Cooke, 2017), Dr Pūras directly calls for a 'paradigm shift' towards the development of culturally appropriate psychosocial interventions as standard practice; working in partnership with people who use mental health services and their carers; respect for diversity, and eliminating coercive treatment and forced confinement.

And, I would add, we need all of this to be backed up by social policy that addresses the root causes of mental distress, such as poverty, discrimination, abuse and structural inequalities.

Dr Pūras also directly addresses the conceptual framework of psychiatry. As I quoted at the start of the chapter, among his report's recommendations are that:

> The urgent need for a shift in approach should prioritize policy innovation at the population level, targeting social determinants and abandon the predominant medical model that seeks to cure individuals by targeting 'disorders'. The crisis in mental health should be managed not as a crisis

of individual conditions, but as a crisis of social obstacles which hinders individual rights. Mental health policies should address the 'power imbalance' rather than 'chemical imbalance'.

There is no question that this report presents those of us working in mental health services, our paymasters, policy makers and governments with an immense challenge. That may be why people in powerful positions seem to have deliberately ignored it. Providing care to people in distress on the basis of this radical demand will entail significant change. Human rights issues are currently largely ignored in our mental health systems, and most services are ill-co-ordinated. Apologists will argue that all the services and benefits called for by critics are currently part of the care offered to clients. The experiences of those who have passed through the system suggest otherwise. And, in any case, if that's true, why do people still complain? We don't need more empty hand-wringing self-justifications; we need reform.

A manifesto for reform

While biomedical research is valuable, we must identify and reject those claims that overstate or misrepresent the evidence base. A dispassionate review of the available evidence supports no longer treating mental health issues as predominantly caused by brain pathology; instead we should recognise that psychological health issues are usually responses to social and environmental factors. This would reduce stigma, more accurately describe the nature of distress, reduce the emphasis on pathology in our mental health discourse, and promote research into and implementation of effective non-biomedical alternatives.

Rather than use medical, pathologising language and methods, we can and should use alternatives that are comprehensible to the ordinary person in the street. To understand and explain our experiences, and to plan services, we need to capture – clearly and objectively – each person's experiences (preferably in their own words) and the circumstances that led to their difficulties. We then need to work together to co-produce plans for what would be of help, and acceptable, to each person. These may include medication but only as part of a package of interventions and support that address their needs. If mental distress is not an illness, why do we need to incarcerate people in hospitals? They could be replaced with residential units designed and managed to operate on a psychosocial model. Current mental health legislation is designed to remove our human rights, even though we retain decision-making capacity. The law must be changed so it respects our rights to make decisions for ourselves unless we are unable to do so and provides for much greater judicial oversight when decisions need to be made on behalf of people who are not able to make decisions for themselves. This means ending the practice whereby doctors are simply empowered to detain and treat people, and instead requires professionals to present evidence to a judge if life-changing decisions need to be made. Human needs are best met by practitioners from a breadth of disciplines and professions, when they are multidisciplinary, democratic and aligned to a psychosocial model. Indeed, psychological health services may be better managed and delivered as social services, alongside other social, community-based, services, not from within the medical system.

One in six working-age adults in England is now taking antidepressant medication, rising to one in five among those aged 65 and over (Duncan & Davis, 2018). The use of antidepressants has doubled in the past 10 years in the UK, as has the average duration of their use. We should not deny the positive role drugs can play but we need to recognise the harms of dependency and withdrawal and put a stop to excessive and unnecessary long-term prescribing. Recent research also shows that long-term use of psychiatric medication leads to poorer outcomes (and can be linked to rising psychological disability). So, doctors should look first to alternatives to medication and prescribing should be short-term, subject to constant review, and always accompanied with a plan for coming off. Those taking medication should be properly and truthfully informed about potential harms as well as benefits, and must no longer be misled by unsubstantiated pseudo-scientific rationales for prescribing, such as brain chemical imbalances.

We must reform the structures of psychological health services themselves. Psychological health care certainly requires appropriate funding, and healthcare professionals will still be needed. But we should not increase funding without systemic reform. We should not fund services with poor outcomes, or assume that current models of leadership, management, governance and service commissioning are always appropriate. Instead, we must prioritise services and treatments that are proven effective, and shift our funding priorities away from fragmented biomedical services to integrated, whole-person, community-based care.

Psychological health problems usually have social or environmental causes. So, psychological health services would most effectively meet our needs if they were able to prioritise prevention and early intervention and were more closely integrated with both physical health services and local authority social, housing and educational services.

We should also reform our public mental health campaigns, avoid using biomedical messages about the causes of mental distress and promote a more psychosocial message about mental health. The general public, the media and mental health professionals need accurate information about the nature, origins and resolution of psychological health issues. We must de-medicalise and de-pathologise public discourse, promote a more constructive and less stigmatising public relationship to psychological difficulties and encourage people to take more active steps to protect and improve their psychological health.

The institutions that uncritically maintain and promote the current, flawed approach to psychological health provision need to be reformed. This may well involve substantial transfers of power – most importantly, from professionals to service users but also from individual clinicians to teams and from psychiatry to others. We must ensure that people who have used services are properly represented on expert groups, and promote a person-centred approach to psychological healthcare that emphasises fundamental human rights and personal autonomy.

Finally, because our mental health – our psychological health – and wellbeing are largely dependent on our social circumstances, and the ways in which we have learned to make sense of, and respond to, challenging life events, we must all work to create a more humane society: to eliminate poverty, especially child poverty, and to reduce financial and social inequality.

This is a manifesto for change. It could even be revolutionary.

References

Allsopp K, Kinderman P (2017). A proposal to introduce formal recording of psychosocial adversities associated with mental health using ICD-10 codes. *The Lancet Psychiatry* 4(9): 664–665.

Boffey D (2015). Prescriptions for Ritalin and other ADHD drugs double in a decade. [Online.] *The Observer*; 15 August.

Cooke A (2017). *Understanding Psychosis and Schizophrenia: why people sometimes hear voices, believe things that others find strange, or appear out of touch with reality... and what can help*. Leicester: British Psychological Society.

Duncan P, Davis N (2018). Four million people in England are long-term users of antidepressants. [Online.] *The Guardian*; 10 August. www.theguardian.com/society/2018/aug/10/four-million-people-in-england-are-long-term-users-of-antidepressants (accessed 25 July 2019).

Kinderman P (2014). *A Prescription for Psychiatry: why we need a whole new approach to mental health and wellbeing*. London: Palgrave Macmillan.

Kinderman P, Allsopp K (2018). Non-diagnostic recording of mental health difficulties in ICD-11. *The Lancet Psychiatry* 5(12): 966.

Pearlson GD, Ford JM (2014). Distinguishing between schizophrenia and other psychotic disorders. *Schizophrenia Bulletin* 40(3): 501–503.

Pūras D (2017). *Report of the Special Rapporteur on the Right of Everyone to the Enjoyment of the Highest Attainable Standard of Physical and Mental Health*. Geneva: Office of the United Nations High Commissioner for Human Rights. http://ap.ohchr.org/documents/dpage_e.aspx?si=A/HRC/35/21

Schwarz A (2015). Still in a crib, yet being given antipsychotics. [Online.] *New York Times*; 10 December.

United Nations (2006). *Convention on the Rights of Persons with Disabilities*. New York, NY: United Nations.

World Health Organization (2018). *International Classification of Diseases* (11th review). Geneva: World Health Organization.

World Health Organization (2012). *WHO QualityRights Tool Kit: assessing and improving quality and human rights in mental health and social care facilities*. Geneva: World Health Organization.

17 | A tale of two tutors: challenging the narrative of diagnosis and disorder in counselling training

Jenny Taper and Jamie-Lee Tipping

At the time of writing this chapter, we were both counsellors and tutors on an integrative counselling degree course.[1] We had become increasingly disheartened by the acceptance in popular thinking of the 'disease model' of human mental and emotional suffering. We believe this view – that appropriate and understandable responses to distressing or traumatic events should be viewed as 'illnesses' or diagnosed as 'disorders' – not only invalidates the experience of the individual but also disempowers and deskills the professionals who work with them. We therefore decided that our first duty as tutors was to ensure that students – the next generation of counsellors – view their future clients not as ill or disordered but as individuals in distress. When they qualify, they will be on the front line, working with clients in distress, and it is therefore crucial that they understand the pressure and further trauma that can be added by a diagnosis.

In this chapter we will share our experience of challenging the disease model of human suffering on our course.

During our own training, we were taught that counsellors were not able to work with clients with a diagnosed psychiatric disorder, as these clients were outside our competency level; we would need to refer them on. This instruction created a distinction between clients experiencing understandable human distress (those we could work with) and clients with a 'disorder' (those we could not work with). Throughout our years of clinical practice, we have come

---

1. We have both since left the university where we delivered the course we describe here, for reasons unrelated to this aspect of our work.

to understand that there is no such distinction, that people's different ways of responding to distress are all understandable if we explore their experiences with them. We have found the starting point with all clients is to ask quite simply, 'What happened to you?' and 'What did you do to survive?'

What surprised us when we trained – and, we believe, many counsellors in training also find it surprising – is that none of the theoretical orientations used by counsellors and psychotherapists actually subscribe to the biomedical model. If we counsellors do not believe that a biomedical model is an explanation of emotional or psychological distress, then should we seek to avoid working with people who have been given these diagnoses? As Carl Rogers said, back in 1976:

> We regard the medical model as an extremely inappropriate model for
> dealing with psychological disturbances. The model that makes more
> sense is a growth model or a developmental model. In other words, we see
> people as having a potential for growth and development and that can
> be released under the right psychological climate. We don't see them as
> sick and needing a diagnosis, a prescription and a cure; and that is a very
> fundamental difference with a good many implications.[2]

We believe that giving labels of 'disorder' to clients can impose a barrier to this exploration of their histories and experiences, invalidate their emotional responses, reframe their creative survival strategies as symptoms of a broken brain and instill a belief that their current distress is evidence of a lifelong illness. We believe that challenging this approach is a prerequisite to developing an effective therapeutic relationship within which the client's experience can be explored, understood and validated as a sane and appropriate response to adversity and trauma.

We therefore made the important decision to challenge the narrative of diagnosis and 'disorder' from the outset in our training, with the aim of breaking the cycle of legitimising psychiatric diagnoses for the next generation of counsellors. As we have said, this shouldn't be so difficult; none of the theoretical models we teach has a biomedical interpretation of human suffering and all of them view change, growth and development as not only possible but the very goal of therapeutic work.

So, why is it so important to place this challenge at the very heart of what we do?

Part of the problem, as we see it, is that the widespread acceptance of constructs such as 'chemical imbalance' in the brain perpetuates the portrayal of people in receipt of a psychiatric diagnosis as different and separate to those

---

2. Carl Rogers, in an interview recorded in 1976 with Professor Anthony Clare on the BBC Radio 4 programme *All in the Mind* (Sanders & Hill, 2014: 60).

without. The oft-quoted 'one in four' statistic relating to incidence of mental 'illness' neatly separates a quarter of the population from the other three-quarters. This perception of 'them and us' leads to the belief that there are people we, as counsellors, can work with and those we cannot. Yet none of us is immune to the emotional toll of adversity, abuse, trauma, loss and discrimination. All of us strive to feel safe and to avoid pain and distress. But the damaging message of 'them and us' has been so well learned that we are not able simply to teach the person-centred theories of change, growth and development and assume that the students will recognise that these theories seek to explain all of human experience. We also need to explicitly challenge 'them and us', 'one in four' and 'diagnosis and disorder' in order to empower our students to be able to see past such unhelpful labels.

What we have realised is that teaching a psychosocial model of understanding is not sufficient to refute the biomedical model, that this needs to be done both implicitly and explicitly within our teaching, and that it must begin from the outset of the students' training.

It is also vital that we have, at the forefront of our minds, our rationale for challenging diagnosis and disorder. We are not seeking to invalidate or deny anyone's individual experience; we need to make clear that, while we do not believe that any individual is 'disordered', we absolutely do believe their distress, their pain and their understandable recourse to survival strategies that may be difficult for some to understand in the absence of context. When challenging the 'broken brain' narrative, we must always offer the alternative understanding – that we are seeking context and meaning in the individual person's experience of distress and that we believe change is possible.

Anyone who has been involved in counselling training at any level will be aware that it is not uncommon for students to have chosen this route of study as a result of their own experiences of distress. More and more often, this will have been 'diagnosed' (often by a GP with a prescription pad) as 'generalised anxiety disorder' or 'depression'. Even more likely to be encountered is the student who has someone close to them who is 'suffering with their mental health'. With this awareness, it would be deeply damaging and possibly counterproductive for us to lead with an attack on the biomedical model.

It is our belief that one of the reasons for the acceptance of psychiatric labelling is that it validates a person's suffering and is experienced by many as the long-sought confirmation that 'something is wrong'; that their difficulties aren't 'all in their head'. Without such a label, the distress may not be, and may not have been, believed.

It is this understanding that has led us to ensure that we only challenge the label when we are confident the student (or client) is able to understand that we do not disbelieve their experience; that we actually wish to further validate and acknowledge their distress by seeking to understand not just what is 'wrong' at the moment, but the history, background and context of what has brought them to this point. With this understanding in place, we then reframe the psychiatric label as a description of current experience that may or may not be useful to the client. When clients know that their distress is not being discounted, when they know that we actually want to understand more and to help them find their own context and meaning, then they may be freed up to share their story without fear of being disbelieved.

It seems to us that this is, in fact, the first task in a trauma-informed practice. The secondary discussion about psychiatric diagnosis having no scientific validity can follow naturally, as the student or client is no longer fearful or defensive. They do not feel they are losing the only thing that validated their experience and can now engage in the debate objectively.

From the very beginning of our course, we place great importance on the language we use to describe and normalise distress. We seek to challenge and reframe pathologising discourse in all of our discussions and interactions. This could be viewed as a key component of the accelerated learning model of teaching to which we adhere – that is, modelling a therapeutic environment and creating a safe space through contracting and setting boundaries. This model of teaching enables students to develop the skills necessary to create such a space for their future clients.

An example of reframing medicalised language is the way in which we challenge the term 'anxiety'. This has come to be viewed as a medical condition or disorder, rather than a normal human emotion. When teaching students about the so-called fight or flight response to a real or perceived threat, we explore the importance of fear in keeping us safe. It becomes clear that fear is a necessary emotion and an appropriate response to danger. By explaining it in this way, we can normalise fear responses to threatening situations. Our individual histories will affect and reinforce how threatening we find a particular situation.

Through class discussion, students connect with the fact that 'anxiety' is a form of fear and is therefore a normal and appropriate response to past and present threats. When a student speaks of 'my anxiety', we respond by asking what is currently leading them to feel anxious. In this way we normalise the feeling and give space for the student to identify the threat, thus underlining the message that anxiousness is a valid response. By reframing 'anxiety' to 'anxiousness', students (and clients) are able to recognise this feeling as an emotion and not a fixed state.

Case studies are a very useful way to further enhance the students' understanding that people with a diagnosed psychiatric disorder are clients with a past history of emotional distress. Case studies offer an opportunity for students to connect to the real-life events and the creative strategies that clients have used/use to survive, cope and function. There are several ways of presenting case studies in teaching, such as watching video clips, creating cases in small groups and reading articles in the counselling literature. Space should be made for students to reflect, unpick and explore the past history of the case study subject, begin to piece together how they developed their creative coping mechanisms and then link this back to what happened to them. Students are asked very early on in training to use case studies as a way of highlighting theory, so this is already a familiar activity, and it later feeds into their learning about psychological formulation. A good example of this would be using the Ted Talk video *The Voices in My Head*, by Eleanor Longden (Longden, 2013).

We use formative case studies and feedback to help students learn to recognise when clients started developing survival strategies to protect themselves from pain and distress. This approach also helps students work out what questions to ask and how to ask them, which they then practise in counselling skills sessions to perfect their use of language and reframing. Constructive feedback after skills practice enables students to attune their approach to ensure they are sensitive to their clients' emotional distress.

Assignments are helpful for us to identify whether students have fully understood the gravitas of what we are teaching them. They are also an opportunity to offer students summative feedback to further enhance their knowledge and point out any areas that we, as tutors, need to revisit in future modules or activities. Therefore, much thought needs to be put into the design and creation of assignment briefs to not only ensure learning outcomes are met but to develop students' ability to gain insight into the client's experience.

As previously mentioned, we teach our students about psychological formulation. To ensure they have understood this, we set an assignment that requires them to pitch the idea for an app that acts as virtual journal for clients to record their story, which can then be shared with other health professionals involved in the client's support. This serves to reduce the number of times clients have to relate what happened to them to all the various professionals they meet. It can also be therapeutic for them to write, and provides the basis for a psychological formulation created jointly by the client and therapist. Students can also add useful additional content to the app, such as techniques, skills and activities. We don't ask them to actually produce the app; we simply use the exercise to encourage them to demonstrate their understanding of the ethical implications and their knowledge of psychological formulation, various interventions and the importance of reducing the client's chances of being re-traumatised through constantly being expected to relive their story.

We have set this assignment twice now, for both full-time and part-time degree students, with some excellent results. We find students become very excited, animated and, more importantly, passionate about the task, especially as the app gives it a contemporary twist. The focus here stays on the client, their journey and their experience of emotional distress – the main point is to not even mention a diagnosis, and the non-pathologising language in the assignment brief encourages the students to work naturally in this way.

Another assignment requires students to conduct a micro-teach in psychological formulation to fellow student counsellors and qualified therapists. This assignment enables students to demonstrate their understanding of the process of psychological formulation and gain a deeper understanding through translating this into a teaching resource. Our aim in using a micro-teach as a form of assessment is to develop the students' confidence in teaching, which in turn cultivates these skills for their future career, which could include facilitating continuing personal development (CPD) events. The assessment process includes feedback sheets for the rest of the group to complete. Following the accelerated learning model, this allows students to have the full experience of delivering a training tool while highlighting the knowledge they have gained in this subject. The summative feedback given by their peers further enhances their training and development skills.

Another exercise we use with students to practise understanding and normalising responses to difficult life situations is to ask them all to complete a Becks Depression Inventory (BDI), imagining they are:

- the mother of a six-week-old baby
- this is her first baby; previously she worked full-time in a professional role
- the baby was distressed during labour and so it was necessary to perform an emergency caesarean section as opposed to the planned natural delivery
- this decision was taken without enough time to administer an epidural and therefore the operation was performed under general anaesthetic
- the baby has colic and cries most of the day
- she is breastfeeding the baby, which she is finding difficult and painful
- the baby wakes to be fed at least twice every night
- her partner took two weeks parental leave but has now returned to work, works long hours and is tired when they get home in the evening.

Through completing the BDI, the students correctly identify that they (in role as this client) may be feeling sad; discouraged about the future; guilty; a failure; disappointed; self-critical; that they are being punished for not being good enough, and tired and irritable. They may derive little satisfaction from the things they do; find it hard to get things done; be worried about their health; have little interest in other people; have difficulty in sleeping; think that their body does not look the way it used to; have lost weight, and have little appetite for food and no interest in sex. They may cry sometimes and might even at times think about suicide.

We then tell them that they all meet the criteria for a diagnosis of 'postnatal depression'.

This is a powerful exercise that illustrates that a diagnosis does nothing more than give a name to a set of completely understandable and appropriate feelings and reactions to difficult circumstances. In this way, students begin to view diagnoses as merely a way of describing current difficulties. Diagnoses are a little like shorthand – it is quicker to say 'postnatal depression' than to list all the thoughts and feelings the client may be experiencing.

Yet even if a psychiatric diagnosis were, indeed, as benign as shorthand or jargon, we would still be justified in claiming that it doesn't serve a helpful purpose for the client; it merely expresses their distress in a different form. We can still say, 'Yes, I agree that this client is distressed, is there a way in which we can help her?'

In practice, though, the diagnosis has named the client as 'mentally ill'. She is now one of 'them', one of the 'one in four'. She is no longer suffering understandable distress while trying to adjust to what may be the biggest change to her role, identity and circumstances she has ever faced. She is no longer struggling to heal from major surgery and overcome a traumatic birth experience, in a state of extreme sleep deprivation and exhaustion, while taking on the total responsibility for the survival of another human being. She is no longer experiencing the loss of status, financial independence and social connection she experienced at work. She is 'ill'.

It is that 'illness' that we are teaching our students to dispute. It's not illness, it's suffering; there is no 'them', there's only 'us'. Our message is yes, of course you can work with this client, and others like her. Most importantly, you can help this client to understand that she was never ill in the first place; she is simply facing understandable challenges and in pain.

This exercise could be done with any psychiatric diagnosis. We chose postnatal depression as it is easily imagined, a 'normal' experience for many women, with easily understandable effects. Some diagnoses describe expressions of distress that may be harder for students to understand or creative survival strategies that we do not often encounter. Some of the events that a client has experienced may be more distressing than we are accustomed to hearing, but the question any counsellor needs always to ask is, 'What happened to you?'

References

Longden E (2013). *The Voices in My Head*. [Video.] Ted2013; February. www.ted.com/talks/eleanor_longden_the_voices_in_my_head?language=en (accessed 24 June 2019).

Sanders P, Hill A (2014). *Counselling for Depression*. London: Sage Publications.

18 Violence under the guise of care: whiteness, colonialism and psychiatric diagnoses

Guilaine Kinouani

Race inequalities within the mental health system are well documented. Black groups are more likely to access mental health care adversely and compulsorily. Further, rates of 'enduring' mental health diagnoses in African-descended people remain higher than in White and Asian groups. In particular, diagnoses of 'schizophrenia' have consistently been found to be elevated in African and Caribbean groups in the UK when compared with their White counterparts (McKenzie & Bhui, 2007; Kirkbride et al, 2012; Bhui et al, 2018).

These enduring inequities have given rise to charges of institutional racism. Over the decades, several theories have been advanced to explain such gross inequities. Few, however, have explored their implications at symbolic-ideological level (Fernando, 2017), the potential role of collective colonial archetypes and the intergenerational context to conceptualise these issues. This chapter proposes a formulation of the experience of a young Black man in a vignette detailing one of my own formative experiences as a mental health professional in London. It will explore the reproduction of imperial configurations and the legacy of colonialism within psychiatric diagnostic practices, using the group-analytic concept of the matrix. Foulkes (1973/1990) defines this as the hypothetical web of communications and relationships that provide the common shared ground that ultimately determines meaning and significance of all events and upon which all communications and interpretations, verbal and non-verbal, rest. To preserve confidentiality, some details have been altered and I have used a pseudonym for the young man.

Levy's story

My first post in the mental health field was as a specialist mental health worker in London. This was in a culturally specific service, staffed by Black workers, that only served people of African and Caribbean heritage. Part of this role included 'key-working' a number of young Black men, most of whom had complex histories and who had typically been diagnosed with 'paranoid schizophrenia'. All had had some contact with the criminal justice system. The vignette concerns one client, let's call him Levy, who was in his early 20s. His support focused on facilitating his 'rehabilitation' into the community and his independence.

Levy was an ambitious, intelligent and charismatic young man, with a history of physical abuse by his father. He did not do well in school and believed his teachers constantly picked on him. Barely out of his teens, Levy had already experienced multiples stop-and-searches by the police. We worked with Levy to co-create a care plan centred on his goals, which were to improve his craft, his rap, and to go to college to pick up where he had left off when he was arrested for smoking joints and subsequently sent to prison. This was where he had become unwell and had been admitted to a medium secure unit under a section 37 of the Mental Health Act (1983).

It had been difficult for us to engage Levy when he was first referred to our service under a Community Treatment Order (CTO), but eventually he became more trusting and open. After six months, his mental health had improved to the point where he repeatedly spoke of wanting to stop his depot medication, a condition of his CTO. The better he got, the more he contested the diagnosis of schizophrenia. He was vocal that his becoming unwell was the result of racism he had experienced in school and at the hands of the police, the pressure he was under at the time, and the cannabis he was smoking to self-medicate.

Levy had got back into college. Things were looking bright. There was a hopeful confidence that his CTO would be lifted at the next review meeting. That day quickly came, and things did indeed look on the up. Initially. Praises were forthcoming from all those involved on his care and support until the White female psychiatrist chairing the meeting asked Levy about 'his schizophrenia'. Levy said he did not have 'schizophrenia'; that he did not believe in 'schizophrenia' and that he did not think it existed. Within seconds, the meeting took a turn for the worse and Levy's section was maintained. The psychiatrist summed up her position as follows: 'Clearly, if you think that there is nothing wrong with you, you are continuing to be a risk to yourself and to others. It seems we have all overestimated the amount of progress that has been made.' Shortly after this statement, the meeting was closed. Within days, Levy's mental health started to deteriorate.

Intersectional vulnerability

The first step in examining Levy's experience is to use intersectional lenses. Doing so allows the spotlight to be placed on the power dynamics at play between Levy and the psychiatrist, and the dynamic of domination this evokes. The term 'intersectionality' (Crenshaw et al, 1995) was coined to conceptualise how systems of oppression (e.g. gender, race, sexuality, class, age, religion, disability) are interconnected, co-constitutive, and give rise to varied patterns of subordination and discrimination. Intersectionality offers an analytic tool to make visible varying patterns of social harm and structural violence. So, for example, the experience of racism of Black women may be compounded by their experience of sexism and/or any other of axes of oppression, and vice versa.

Similarly, the gendered nature of racism will mean that the intersection of Blackness and maleness will evoke different social scripts, stereotypes and tropes and, therefore, trigger different systemic responses and experiences of discrimination to the intersection of Blackness and femaleness. Levy is a young Black man from inner-city London, who has been convicted of a drug-related offence, has been sectioned under the Mental Health Act (1983) and has been given a diagnosis of 'paranoid schizophrenia'. Race, gender, class, age, inner-city background are all colliding factors here, laying out Levy's structural experiences. Cumulatively, they function as a catalyst for his detention, diagnosis, pathway onto the mental health system and the psychiatrist's perceptions of him.

Through much of his existence, Levy was exposed to constant reminders of his presumed dangerousness and deviance – a gendered and racialised stereotype through which his everyday reality was experienced, as illustrated by the stop-and-searches he was routinely subjected to. Such experiences would have likely reinforced his distrust for authority figures – arguably, an adaptive response to the trauma of oppression. Levy's structural trauma intersects with his interpersonal trauma – his possible sense of powerlessness and subjugation have been compounded by his father's abuse. Through these lenses, Levy's contestation of the diagnosis of 'schizophrenia' and his suspicion towards diagnostic categories may be interpreted as an act of resistance – a rejection of the pathologisation of his lived experience; an attempt to reclaim power by self-defining in a social context where submissiveness and subservience have been set as normative for him.

The need to be heard

Levy is craving to speak. His choice of artistic expression reflects this need. Rap is a means for Levy to express himself and expressing himself keeps him well. Despite his history of structural and interpersonal trauma, Levy has regained a sense of hope and has committed to a new start, largely on his own terms. Rap links Levy to his West African ancestry and its oral tradition. Connection seems an important theme in his 'recovery'. There is, at least symbolically, a reconnection with his roots; perhaps, too, a wish to connect to his history, to reconnect to the world; perhaps to connect to himself. Levy's artistic choice thus parallels his emancipatory efforts and may, at its most fundamental level, represent the need to be heard and feel connected.

Dismissing him in the present context forces a disconnection. Further, it echoes previous trauma and closely reproduces his adverse life experiences of being at the receiving end of abuses of power (paternal abuse, police profiling, volatile and possibly biased relationships with teachers). It reconfirms his experience of authority figures as figures of distrust and brutality, which may be triggering if not re-traumatising for him. Thus, forcing a diagnosis of 'schizophrenia' onto Levy is another abuse of power. Confining him within a 'mentally ill' or 'schizophrenic' identity and discourse under the pretext of increasing his 'insight' and thus allegedly reducing the risks he poses to self and/or others is a premise with very little empirical support. It is one that may, in fact, be increasing risks to him (Misdrahi, Denard & Courtet, 2011). It is also forcing a Eurocentric conceptualisation and a medical explanatory model onto him. This everyday practice is disturbing. Levy has the capacity and fundamental right to define his experience otherwise. And, indeed, he has chosen to do so.

The unconscious reproduction of colonial configurations

Any meeting of individuals is a microcosm of society and a sample of power relations of the wider social world. The functioning of any group consequently reflects the functioning of society (Hopper & Weinberg, 2017). Similarly, the mind of an individual speaks something of their wider social context. The group analytic concept of the matrix may help to illuminate such collective processes and the reproduction of colonial configurations within this vignette. Foulkes, the founder of group analysis, was among the first Western scholars to highlight the importance of the social to the psychological and to locate individuals and their relational interactions within their socio-political, economic and historical contexts (Foulkes, 1973/1990). The group matrix, one of his theoretical conceptualisations of interpersonal relationships, remains a core tenet of group analysis.

Foulkes describes it as the intersubjective field within which the group operates, a 'field effect', primarily unconscious, which interconnects all people in a network in which they 'meet, communicate and interact' (Foulkes & Anthony, 1957/1984: 26). The group matrix gives meaning to all human communications and, indeed, without it, our understanding of our interactions can only be incomplete. More contemporary groups analysts have come to formulate the matrix as a tri-partite interconnected entity incorporating the personal matrix, the dynamic matrix and the foundation matrix (Hopper & Weinberg, 2017).

The personal matrix contains the more idiosyncratic aspects of our selves – for example, our psychological traits, relational history, our 'object relations'. Levy's history of paternal abuse would feature at this level. The dynamic matrix encapsulates the interpersonal communication and interactions happening in the here and now between people in any setting. Interactions between Levy and the psychiatrist, or between the staff and Levy and all those engaged in the review meeting, would be situated at this level. The foundation matrix is concerned with more distal or structural, communicational arrangements rooted in history and already in place, such as social structures and institutions. Of particular interest here would be the service that supports Levy, psychiatry as an institution and the socio-political context. All of these are located in the foundation matrix.

A final crucial aspect of the group matrix is the social unconscious. The social unconscious is taken to refer to internalised social configurations and to the properties of the social world that evade our conscious awareness (Hopper & Weinberg, 2017). It has been conceptualised as the co-constructed shared unconscious of members of a particular social system such as community, society, nation or culture. It can be unclear in Foulkes' writing at what level the social unconscious sits in the group matrix. Nonetheless, it has since been suggested that the distinction between the social and the psychological, and therefore between the foundation and personal matrix, is illusory (Dalal, 2001).

One way to conceptualise the continuing presence of the past in the present and, with that, the reproduction of colonial configurations, is through the concept of equivalence. In the same way that individuals tend to recreate past situations, particularly those within which they have been traumatised, we are equally compelled to unconsciously transfer past social arrangements onto present situations and thus create equivalences, or group transferences (Hopper & Weinberg, 2017). It is notable that Levy's treatment does have strong echoes of the past. The imposition of the psychiatric diagnosis of 'schizophrenia' is indeed evocative of colonial configurations and arrangements, and this needs attention. That there may thus be unconscious social and historical scripts that shape and give meaning to our relational patterns is not a new idea. This group analytic concept, however, is rarely used as a prism to examine race inequalities within the mental health system and diagnostic practices. The remainder of this chapter will attempt to do so.

Psychiatric diagnoses as epistemic violence

Levy's intersectional positioning disadvantages him epistemically and renders him vulnerable to epistemic violence. Epistemic violence is a term used by postcolonial scholars to refer to the construction of the Other by Western thinkers and philosophers. According to Spivak (1991), epistemic violence is a process by which non-Western methods or approaches to knowledge and their worldviews are obstructed. Spivak posits that imperialist subjugation of non-Western understanding, or the 'Othering' of the colonial subject's mode of knowing/being and, more generally, that of those who are at the bottom of social hierarchies – the 'subaltern' – has been central to the colonial project. This dynamic is said to represent attempts at erasing the consciousness of the Other and replacing it with Western knowledges. In that sense, we may say it reproduces whiteness.

Whiteness may be conceptualised as the production and reproduction of the dominance and superiority of people socially racialised as White (Green,

Sonn & Matsebula, 2007). It is the cause of ongoing race inequality and power differentials between various racial groups and White people and the origin of specific patterns of social relations within particular spatial contexts (Neely & Samura, 2011). Whiteness holds much of its power by the ways in which it has become woven into the very fabric of Western societies and normalised, so that all aspects of these cultures, norms and values centre and privilege White people, their worldview, experience of the world and ways of making sense of the same.

Seen from this perspective, Levy refuses to subscribe to a medical, supposedly objective reading of his experience – a reading that is consistent with a White Eurocentric belief system and thus normalises whiteness. However, Levy's worldview and knowledge is disappeared in the way that epistemic violence seeks to disappear 'Other' knowledge (Spivak,1991). The concept of dormant racism proposes that much invisible racial prejudice lurks, inactive or implicit, within both the social and the individual unconscious, until the conditions for its externalisation are met. Usually these come in the form of challenges to White normative expectations or threats to the social order (Kinouani, 2015). Levy's direct challenge to psychiatric discourses constitutes just such a threat and may be interpreted as a socially transgressive act. Levy refuses to stay in his place. He is refusing to bow down to a socially authoritative figure. He is effectively challenging the authority of the Master.

Self-definition is the quintessential act of liberation for colonised bodies. By seeking to define themselves, the colonised seek to reject the inferiority, pathology and/or dysfunction that has been located inside them and thereby reclaim bodily and psychic autonomy (Fanon, 1952). A large body of evidence suggests African-descended people are much less likely to use biomedical lenses to make sense of their distress (Degnan et al, 2018; Fernando, 2010, 2017). Many have criticised psychiatric diagnoses for their conceptual and empirical limitations as well as their potential to be weaponised as tools of oppression and discrimination (Fernando, 2010, 2017; Johnstone & Boyle, 2018). Further, numerous calls have been made for a nuanced framing of the concept of 'insight', taking into careful consideration cultural beliefs, explanatory models and social context. Yet Levy's challenge cannot be tolerated by the psychiatrist. How dare he speak?

The implicit outrage in this context is racialised and has imperialist resonance that is evocative of the social unconscious. The whole Black support team and its collective voice are swiftly discredited, albeit more covertly. All of us are infantilised and, together with Levy, positioned as non-knowers. In other words, we are not afforded epistemic credibility. In the words of the psychiatrist, as chair: 'We have all overestimated that amount of progress that has been made.' Thus, the psychiatrist's opinion is presented as a collective voice, a consensus. However, this position is arrived at without seeking the views or opinions of anyone else in the room. The diagnosis is the truth and it trumps all. The Black team's voice is immaterial; it can be silenced and also disappeared.

Silencing and invisibilisation

As Levy is considered to be incapable of speaking for himself, his body can be controlled via an extension of his CTO, which, incidentally, comes with compulsory pharmacological treatment, in order to manage purported risks. The Black team, as Others, are not expected to speak reason either, and so can be spoken for by the psychiatrist. The assessment of Levy as 'a risk to himself and to others' is unjustifiable in view of the evidence presented and of his index offence. But Levy is any event 'wrong' in contesting the very existence of 'schizophrenia', which provides further evidence 'that there is something wrong' with him. And that something is called 'paranoid schizophrenia'. The risks Black men present are systematically overestimated and the structural violence and trauma they experience are systematically underestimated, invisibilised or erased.

In this vignette, the psychiatrist becomes the guardian of society's safety and, more subtly, morality. In the dynamic matrix, the silencing of Levy as a Black subject maintains the fantasy of Eurocentric universalism and superiority. Levy has been colonised. He becomes a passive object for the production of racialised imagery. This passivity is reproduced by his care team. We all sit in silence as the CTO is renewed. I feel distraught but dare not speak. I doubt my own expertise and credibility. I feel rage at the injustice, and perhaps the others do too but are keeping quiet, waiting for someone else in the team, perhaps a more senior colleague, to speak, to add weight to Levy's challenge.

No one does. Perhaps a bystander effect takes hold. The silence continues after the meeting ends. The issues are never raised. This may be due to shame or to guilt. Perhaps it is a collective sense of helplessness. Levy disengages from the team and, shortly after, becomes unwell. What or who is responsible for Levy's deterioration? Is it the disconnection or splitting from his reality that he is forced to experience? Is it the so-called paranoid schizophrenia? Is it an ontological malaise? Is it the structural racism contained within the epistemic imposition of the diagnosis? Is it the trauma of a further act of subjugation that perhaps hooked onto or activated prior deep and unresolved wounds located in his personal matrix? Is it the gagging of Levy and the smothering of his need to speak and be heard? Is it the introjection of the disturbance that has been and continues to be located in him? Is it the intergenerational baggage Levy is carrying alone? Is it a legitimate sense of betrayal?

Silence can be collusion. It is often denial. Silence can be the wilful refusal to confront distressing situations and an attempt to avoid conflicts. Silence can also hide intergenerational trauma and historical terror. The fear of challenging the powerful Master and their 'superior' knowledge is a historical configuration that is likely located in our social unconscious. So too is the fear of naming whiteness and thus challenging the status quo. These fears are nevertheless associated with structural consequences within the foundation 'level' of the matrix, such as threats to the continuity of funding and, consequently, increased risks of ontological precariousness for the Black organisation. Such material concerns mirror the fear of annihilation or destruction that whiteness projects onto the Black psyche via control of its body.

Perhaps all those fears are silently in operation in the room and within all of us. Stobo (2005) proposes that silence serves to regulate and maintain a psychic equilibrium and that the space between Black and White people holds the fear of something that cannot be spoken – specifically, our shared histories of imperialism, colonialism and enslavement. Stobo thus suggests that part of what is feared and difficult to articulate is a discovery or acknowledgement of racism. This unexpressed conflict, she posits, manifests as a disturbance that is located in certain bodies – ideally, those racialised as Black, onto whom a pathology becomes necessarily located. Here, it is Levy's body that carries the bulk of the violence of whiteness, but the Black team is equally exposed to trauma. One may say they are powerlessly witnessing a symbolic lynching scene, knowing they too could suffer such fate. The collective intergenerational trauma of White violence is reproduced under the guise of care.

Concluding thoughts

The collective trauma of our imperial past is still to be resolved. This vignette offers a framework to reflect on how colonial configurations may be reproduced within psychiatry and specifically here, within diagnostic practices via collective and social unconscious mechanisms. The influence of the past through the mapping of the different 'levels' of the analytic group matrix proposes that colonialism and imperialism are alive within us, between us and within social structures. Some of us may be more intersectionally vulnerable to its violence. Spivak (1991) has asked, 'Can the subaltern speak?' In the present case, the clear answer is no. The imposition of the psychiatric diagnosis has denied the young, Black, male, poor, uneducated, 'mad' and 'bad' subaltern the right to speak, to be listened to and to recover agency over his own body by making self-alienation and splitting conditions of his freedom and by enacting epistemic violence. In doing so, it has stripped Levy of his subjecthood and reproduced interpersonal, structural and intergenerational trauma. Not only for Levy and for the Black staff involved but collectively for all those who continue to suffer whiteness-related brutality.

Acknowledgements

This is for the young Black men deprived of their liberty primarily because they are young, Black men. Thank you to Amamassa Kpognon, for your insightful contributions in the early draft of this chapter.

References

Bhui K, Halvorsrud K, Rhodes J, Nazroo J, Francis J (2018). *The Impact of Racism on Mental Health*. Briefing paper. London: The Synergi Collaborative Centre.

Crenshaw K, Gotanda N, Peller G, Thomas K (eds) (1995). *Critical Race Theory: the key writings that formed the movement*. New York, NY: The New Press.

Dalal F (2001). The social unconscious: a post-Faulknerian perspective. *Group Analysis 34*(4): 539–555.

Degnan A, Berry K, James S, Edge D (2018). Development, validation and cultural-adaptation of the knowledge about psychosis questionnaire for African Caribbean people in the UK. *Psychiatry Research 263*:199-206.

Fanon F (1952). *Black Skin, White Masks* (Markmann CL, trans). New York, NY: Grove Press.

Fernando S (2017). *Institutional Racism in Psychiatry and Clinical Psychology: race matters in mental health*. London: Palgrave Macmillan.

Fernando S (2010). *Mental Health, Race and Culture* (3rd ed). London: Red Globe Press.

Foulkes SH (1973/1990). The group as a matrix of the individual's mental life. Republished in: Foulkes E (ed) (1990). *Selected Papers of SH Foulkes: psychoanalysis and group analysis*. London: Karnac Books (pp223–233).

Foulkes SH, Anthony EJ (1957/1984). *Group Psychotherapy: the psychoanalytical approach*. London: Karnac Books.

Green MJ, Sonn CC, Matsebula J (2007). Reviewing whiteness: theory, research, and possibilities. *South African Journal of Psychology 37*(3): 389–419.

Hopper E, Weinberg H (2017). *The Social Unconscious in Persons, Groups, and Societies. Volume 3: the foundation matrix extended and re-configured*. London: Karnac Books.

Johnstone L, Boyle M, with Cromby J, Dillon J, Harper D, Kinderman P, Longden E, Pilgrim D, Read J (2018). *The Power Threat Meaning Framework: towards the identification of patterns in emotional distress, unusual experiences and troubled or troubling behaviour, as an alternative to functional psychiatric diagnosis*. Leicester: British Psychological Society.

Kinouani G (2015). *Black deference and dormant racism: the politics of knowing one's place*. [Blog.] Race Reflections. https://racereflections.co.uk/2015/08/04/black-deference-or-and-dormant-racism-the-politics-of-knowing-ones-place (accessed 29 June 2019).

Kirkbride JB, Errazuriz A, Croudace TJ et al (2012). Incidence of schizophrenia and other psychoses in England, 1950–2009: a systematic review and meta-analyses. *PLoS One 7*(3). https://journals.plos.org/plosone/article?id=10.1371/journal.pone.0031660

McKenzie K, Bhui K (2007). Institutional racism in mental health care. *British Medical Journal 334*: 649.

Misdrahi D, Denard S, Courtet P (2011). Insight and schizophrenia: what roles in the suicide risk? *Annales Médico-psychologiques revue psychiatrique 169*(7): 426-428.

Neely B, Samura M (2011). Social geographies of race: connecting race and space. *Ethnic and Racial Studies 34*(11): 1933–1952.

Spivak GC (1991). Can the subaltern speak? In: Nelson C, Grossberg L (eds). *Marxism and the Interpretation of Culture*. Urbana: University of Illinois Press (pp1–15).

Stobo B (2005). *Location of disturbance with a focus on race, difference and culture*. Dissertation submitted in partial fulfilment of the Masters in Group Analysis, London: Birkbeck College.

19 | Names matter, language matters, truth matters[1]

Jacqui Dillon

What I want to do here is think about language and mental health and how our use of language – the words we use to describe people – is an insidious way of changing the way we think about people. I believe that what we are doing when we use medicalised language is rendering intelligible things unintelligible and that is a deliberate ploy that happens throughout psychiatry. One of the things we can do as activists, survivors and practitioners, which is quite radical but quite subtle, is to use ordinary human language to describe extraordinary human experiences.

For me language shapes the way we think about ourselves. There's a lot written about this – for example, Einstein wrote a really interesting paper about language and mentality in which he argues that 'the mental development of the individual and his way of forming concepts depend to a high degree upon language' (Einstein, 1941/42). What I want to do here is focus down on language and the ways in which psychiatry uses it to colonise the way we think about ourselves and each other.

Judith Herman's wonderful book *Trauma and Recovery* (1992) was given to me when I'd not long come out of psychiatric hospital. I'd been admitted to hospital when my daughter was a toddler and, like many survivors of bad things that happen to us in childhood, including sexual abuse, the experience of being a

---

1. This chapter is based on Jacqui Dillon's presentations at the 'A Disorder for Everyone!' events in London on 6 September 2018 and Edinburgh on 28 September 2018.

parent brought up for me tons of stuff that happened in my childhood. It's a very common and understandable thing to happen. For me, as a survivor of organised, ritualised abuse throughout my childhood that I'd never disclosed to anybody, the birth of my daughter was the most incredible, wonderful experience; the first time I'd ever felt proud of myself. I'd been able to give birth to this perfect baby. But within days this idyllic scene was invaded by demons from my past and I began to have these absolutely devastating, terrifying experiences.

One of the ways I survived as a child was that I'd managed to keep the abuse that happened to me separate, in another world. I think lots of children do this. Dissociation is still not understood properly and acknowledged for how important it is. I had this public world where everything was OK and I had this private world where horror happened, and when I became a mother it was much harder to keep them apart. So they ended up colliding in this catastrophic way, and I ended up as a psychiatric patient.

The first person I tried to tell about some of the things that happened to me as a baby was a psychiatrist. Bear in mind that the people who abused me, like many who abuse children on an industrial scale, were very sophisticated in grooming and terrorising children to ensure we didn't speak. I had been terrorised; I'd been told that if I told about it, I would be killed; that people wouldn't believe me; that people would think I was mad and I'd be locked up. These are very powerful and frightening things to say to a child. And then, when I ended up in psychiatric hospital, guess what – the things that my abusers said would happen happened to me. I was not believed. I was told I was mad, that I was 'delusional'. In fact, the psychiatrist I told this to, said, 'Jacqui, we have lots of people in here who describe these kinds of experiences and when we get their families in and we all talk about it together, they realise this is just part of their illness.' And I remember one of the voices that I heard at that time saying to me, 'Pick up that filing cabinet and drop it on his head.'

Fortunately, I didn't do that, or I'd still be banged up in a secure unit. Another of my voices said to me, 'Get out of the room.' And I got out of the room, which is good, because if I'd stayed, I would have lost it and got myself into very serious trouble. I walked down the corridor and I went into the bathroom and into a cubicle and I smashed my head against the wall. The horror and outrage of having the words of my abusers reiterated to me by the people who were meant to be offering me support was absolutely devastating. And I am still furious about it, because it happens to people all the time and it's wrong. It's so wrong.

What's underneath that anger is my heartbreak at the way this society, all Western societies, treats people who have already suffered enough. What the psychiatric system does is cause more harm, iatrogenic harm. It robs us of our autonomy, deprives us of our liberty, forces psychiatric medications on us that we don't want to take, and goes on making us take them even when we leave hospital, and for the rest of our lives. And they do this under the guise of the so-called bio-medical model, which I think should have been consigned to the dustbin many years ago, because all it does is cause people harm while simultaneously creating a lot of profit for the people who make these drugs. We have a system that causes more harm to people who are already suffering and profits from that suffering, and that sickens me. At the heart of my anger is the heartbreak of meeting people who have been told lies – hypotheses as if they're facts – about what's wrong with them and how these drugs will help, and have had their lives ruined by this.

A psychiatrist who doesn't do this is the wonderful Judith Herman. My therapist handed her book to me. I'd been out of hospital a few months and was lucky enough to find a therapist who did believe me, who did believe that people do terrible things to children and who also believed that people are more than the terrible things that happened to them, which for me was like finding gold. What people want is to be believed and acknowledged. It's that simple. Except it's not that simple because, if psychiatrists did believe them and acknowledge their needs, they'd have to design services to meet those needs, rather than the system we've got, which doesn't want to hear about people's suffering and doesn't want to address the epidemic of child abuse in this country or the epidemics of social inequality, racism, poverty, social exclusion – all those issues that research tells us drives people mad.

One of the things I have come to recognise is that psychiatry is a system that we, as a society, have put in place to keep away the people we decide are mad, and psychiatrists are the gatekeepers. And psychiatry is operating within a neoliberal system that makes money out of people's suffering and doesn't want to engage with their suffering because, if we did, it would mean a revolution.

One of the things that Judith Herman does in the first part of her book is an analysis of trauma – the way trauma throughout history has been acknowledged and then, because it's inconvenient, gets buried – much in the same as it does at an individual level. She talks about the First World War, when many of those young men came back traumatised from their war experiences and were diagnosed with shell shock – until it became inconvenient for the government, who needed them to return to the front line, and told them if they didn't go back, they would be court martialed. And even after the war, people with shell shock were told there was nothing wrong with them, or it wasn't caused by their exposure to shelling in the trenches, because that would have entitled them to war benefits.

So, this is a good example of what the authorities do: they blame you for your circumstances because it's politically inconvenient to acknowledge your reality.

So, when the first part of Judith Herman's book talks about the way society systematically does that, for me, that was really important, as someone who had just come out of psychiatric hospital. I was feeling pretty mad, I was hearing terrifying voices, I felt very suicidal and paranoid, I was cutting myself on a regular basis, I was seeing things, I was hearing things, I was having lots of frightening things happening to me, but for me the most crazy-making thing was someone telling me that what was happening to me was because I was born with a biological illness. I mean, how fucking crazy-making is that? I am sitting there, telling him these horrific things happened to me, which if they happened to anyone would be deeply affecting, and this psychiatrist was saying to me, ' No, those things didn't happen to you, you've got this other thing and here's this label that we are going to stick on you.' That is going to make me feel sane? I don't think so.

Recovery without psychiatry

People say to me, 'When you came out of hospital, how did you recover?' And I say, 'Without psychiatry.' And that is totally true and a sad indictment of our mental health services, because that's what happened when I got out of the psychiatric system. When I stopped allowing them to define my reality, when I found what I call an empathic witness who would walk alongside me and bear witness to what happened to me, for the first time I got to speak my truth in the presence of another who was committed to hearing my truth.

In the second part of the book, Judith Herman outlines how we help people who have been deeply traumatised. She describes a number of ways but for me one of the most important ones is that we establish safety with people. I do a lot of consultancy work with mental health trusts and, when I work with their psychosis teams, I'm amazed that literally, the moment someone enters their service, they are talking about a discharge plan. How unwelcoming is that? Obviously we don't want people to become institutionalised but, when someone is in a very frightened state, when they are remembering in a metaphorical way the worst things that ever happened to them, they are in significant crisis, and we are talking about getting them out of the service immediately, rather than making them feel welcome and giving them some time. What people need is time. I was subjected to 10 years of organised abuse. How are six sessions of CBT meant to reach that?

What people need is long-term therapeutic relationships. You need time to get to know and trust somebody. You need time to start remembering and disclosing things, because the thing about trauma is that the memories don't come back in an organised, linear manner. They come back in ways that are quite fragmented and what helps is the relationship, I believe. John Bowlby, the father of attachment theory, says the human psyche is like the human skeleton – it has the capacity to heal in the same way that a bone does when we break it – the mind and body will galvanise and want to heal it, and the same is true of the human psyche (Bowlby, 1988). And one of the things that upsets me the most is the way biological psychiatry completely interrupts that natural healing process. If they just left people alone, it would do less harm to them than telling people the bullshit they do.

So, Judith Herman writes about the importance of safety, remembrance and mourning for what is lost when you are recovering from trauma – and that can take time. For people like me, who have been utterly betrayed by the people who are meant to be protecting you, you may need to do a lot of testing of this relationship with the therapist. Is this person really safe? Are they going to be able to see who I am? Are they really going to be able to bear to hear what I have to say to them? Are they going to be able to see beyond all this distress that I am currently experiencing to who I really am? You go from feeling nothing, from these very numbed-out states, to feeling flooded with emotions you don't understand. You vacillate between these states. And for me, what is different when you have a therapeutic alliance, an empathic witness, a safe space, is that you begin to feel the feelings in connection to the actual events, to the real losses, and that is when the healing occurs, because you feel the feelings of grief, loss, rage, disgust, horror, whatever it is, in a way that makes sense. And for me that is wholly contingent on having a healing relationship, because most the traumas I am talking about were interpersonal violations, so the only thing that could help was a healing interpersonal relationship, in my experience.

The final thing that Herman talks about is reconnection with community and society. And again, what I see happening in services is we get people into hospital, we do no work with them whatsoever, we get them 'stabilised' – ie. we put them on medication so they're not annoying us anymore – we don't care about what effects that medication has – too bad, you're ill, you've got to keep taking it – and then we say, 'Right, you are in recovery now.' And you say, 'I feel worse, actually. I feel really bad. I don't make sense to myself.' Now to me that's insight. It's not buying the bullshit psychiatrists tell you about yourself. Real insight is when your experiences make sense to you and you can explain them to yourself and your emotional state makes sense to you.

If I'm walking down the street and suddenly I get flooded with emotion, I'll think, 'What is going on here?' And then I'll think, 'Ah, that man – his breath smells of vodka and that reminds me of a time when I was younger,' and that makes sense to me. It doesn't mean I'm not affected by what's happening, but I'll know why I'm suddenly feeling that way. But if I spoke to a mental health practitioner who subscribes to the biomedical model, they'd say, 'Oh, that's an olfactory delusion.' Right. That's fucking helpful. So, what they've done is mystify my experience. They've given it some fancy-dancy label and now I've not got any idea what was happening to me. But if we talk in very ordinary terms, it restores meaning.

What we are, we human beings, is sense-making beings. What we want is to be able to understand ourselves in our world around us. But none of that happens in the psychiatric system. They say, 'You're in recovery now. We've taken down the Community Mental Health Team sign and we're now a Recovery Service; we do recovery.' And when I read Judith Herman's work 20-odd years ago, recovery was a really radical idea. But now, like many things, because it's a good idea, the biomedical model has colonised it. So, what they mean by recovery now is that you are a good patient, you are a compliant patient and, because it's politically expedient, you need to get your arse out of here, get off benefits and get a fucking job. Even though there are no jobs or there are zero-hour contract jobs and, even though, for a lot of people, they'll be better off and have more security on benefits, it doesn't matter.

They talk about people recovering but they've done no actual work with them. They've done nothing to try to understand why this crisis has occurred, why they've been suffering so much, why they are having these experiences, what is really going on, how they can make what's happening meaningful to them so they can really learn from this crisis, this terrible emergence of all of this suffering and pain. Because I believe it is always meaningful, that it is possible to co-create some meaning out of what is happening to them and the person can gain some strength from that. But that rarely happens unless you are fortunate enough to find someone who doesn't subscribe to the biomedical ways of thinking about people that dominate the psychiatric system.

Another of the things Judith Herman writes about that has been really crucial to my work is this idea of finding a survivor mission. She says that when you have been subject to horrific things and then you go to services that cause you more harm, often that leaves you feeling really, really angry. Then you get told you've got anger issues. Fuck off! I interviewed a woman called Audrey from Glasgow for a book I co-edited called *Living with Voices* (Romme et al, 2009). She had been sexually abused as a child and ended up in the psychiatric system and she was very, very angry because she understood, even in her very distressed state, that this was what was causing her distress – that she had been abused as a little girl. She was understandably angry about being sectioned, having her liberty taken away from her, being forced to take medication that she didn't want to take, and that all her attempts to talk about the things that were making her crazy were, in her words, 'punished'. Her meds would be increased and her leave would be withdrawn because she was trying to deal with things inside. She was a young woman, about 20 years of age, and she got referred for anger management classes, and I said, 'What did you feel about that,' and she said, 'Fucking furious,' which to me was a wholly appropriate response.

What mental health services are most frightened of are people's emotions – their own and other people's. 'The team's feeling very anxious and we feel this person should have their medication increased,' they say. So? So, perhaps the team needs some medication?

Judith Herman says it's entirely appropriate for people to feel angry about the things that have happened to them. When you have been subject to violations, injustices, whatever words you want to use, it's entirely appropriate to feel angry about it. To me, feeling angry is like saying, 'I matter. You've treated me badly and I'm not having that.' It's a really appropriate response.

And what Judith Herman says is it's really important for survivors to find a vehicle for their rage because, for many of us who were brought up in dysfunctional families, what we learned is that anger is scary, it's toxic, it's harmful. For me, there was a time when I was quite frightened of my anger and for years, when I'd feel angry with someone, because I didn't feel able to express that for lots and lots of reasons – I didn't feel entitled, I was scared of them retaliating, I didn't have a voice – I'd go off and hurt myself. It was something I learned as a very small child. And it was only through the process of therapy that I began to recognise that when people hurt my feelings, offended me, said things that were really outrageous, I would hurt myself. I remember that dawning realisation through the process of being in a therapeutic relationship and, as I began to appreciate it, I thought, 'Fuck that for a game of soldiers, I need to learn how to start asserting myself.' I still remember the very first time after that, when someone said something that really hurt my feelings and really hurt me, when previously I would have taken it out on myself, I remember actually articulating it. I said, 'I'm not OK with what you've just said,' and my voice said, 'Yes, you tell them!', and that was a massive turning point. I began to recognise that anger is incredibly powerful and an incredible motivator and it's that anger that has enabled me to become an activist to try to change how people think about these experiences, because it breaks my heart.

At its root, I believe that, whatever has happened to them, people can be OK again. And that is one of the things that disgusts me most about the biomedical model – how pessimistic it is about people. It has such little faith in people's capacities to heal from terrible experiences and that to me is a travesty. We don't hear enough stories about how, even though someone has been subject to horrific experiences, with an empathic witness, with time, with space, with an opportunity to make sense of things, they do recover. Because the mind and body are entirely geared up to heal, so all we have to do is make space for that. One of the things my first therapist used to say to me is, 'My job is akin to a midwife – actually what has happened within you is an entirely natural process and my job is to be here to help you like a midwife. A midwife doesn't make a baby new born; our body knows what to do. Sometimes it might get a bit stuck and need a bit of guidance but essentially our bodies know what to do.' And the same is true of healing, I believe. That has been both my own experience and that of many, many people I've supported.

So, finding this survivor mission for many of us is about taking social action. It's a willingness to speak the unspeakable. I see my work as a form of social justice because, like the saying goes, those who forget the past are condemned to repeat it (Santayana, 2016). It's not about revenge and it's not about seeking compensation. This took me a long time to realise. Even if I were given a zillion pounds, no one could give me back the childhood that was stolen from me; nothing can change what's happened, apart from healing. The bottom line is, I still feel robbed of a secure childhood, which literally impacts every aspect of your experience. But what I think a survivor mission and the choice to speak out is actually about is trying to transcend your suffering now you've had enough empathy, enough witnessing, and make it a gift to other people.

Doublethink

This is another really important quote from Judith Herman. She says:

> The psychological distress symptoms of traumatized people simultaneously
> call attention to the existence of an unspeakable secret and deflect
> attention from it. This is most apparent in the way traumatized people
> alternate between feeling numb and reliving the event. The dialectic
> of trauma gives rise to complicated, sometimes uncanny alterations of
> consciousness, which George Orwell, one of the committed truth-tellers of
> our century, called 'doublethink', and which mental health professionals,
> searching for calm, precise language, call 'dissociation'. (Herman, 1992: 1–2)

This is a really powerful quote on a number of different levels in terms of thinking about what Herman calls the dialectic of trauma. This is where traumatised people are simultaneously calling attention to the existence of something terrible that has happened to them while deflecting attention from it by something like self-injury, and professionals get very caught up with the coping mechanism, rather than what actually might be driving it.

Let's face it, we are living in a dystopian universe right now, and I want to extend this idea of doublethink so we are not just talking about the ways in which traumatised people survive traumatic experiences. Doublethink operates on a number of different levels. It comes from George Orwell's book *Nineteen Eighty-Four* (1949) and it's defined as 'the act of ordinary people simultaneously accepting two mutually contradictory beliefs as correct, often in distinct social contexts' (McArthur, 1992).

So, in this dystopian world that Orwell was writing about in *Nineteen Eighty-Four*, they had to use this doublethink. So, war is peace, freedom is slavery, ignorance is strength – these absolutely contradictory statements which they had to hold as fact in their minds at the same time. And of course, it's the opposite to cognitive dissonance, because with cognitive dissonance there's an awareness that the two contradict each other, whereas doublethink is distinguished by the lack of cognitive dissonance: the person is completely unaware of any conflict or contradiction.

This often happens in psychiatric contexts, and it can happen in families too. So, for example, in psychiatric settings, I've heard statements like; 'It would not surprise me if such abuse greatly worsens the psychopathology of a child already in the early stages of the illness.'

The number of care planning and other meetings I've been to where you hear this kind of statement. One woman I knew who had been through years and years of hideous abuse – childhood abuse, torture, sexual abuse; she'd been trafficked, domestic violence, a catalogue of awful traumas. She went to see a psychiatrist and I went to support her and she was describing her experiences to him and he said:

'It's awful you were raped throughout your childhood, and then you were put into care and you were sexually abused in care, and I know you got a lot of racist abuse and you were very poor and you got into that domestic violence and you had your children taken away from you and now you've got schizophrenia, poor thing.' And I say, 'For a seemingly intelligent person, how is it possible that you can hold those two things separately in your mind?' It's a rhetorical question. I know the answer. It's because of the privileging of biology over everything else.

People recount these awful histories and what they are told is that they've got a 'personality disorder', which for me is such an insult. That's when I look to people like Mary Boyle, who writes:

> It is no wonder that psychiatry is fearful of context and has to devise so many strategies to avoid it, because context constantly threatens to make emotional and behavioural problems intelligible or, to put it another way, it threatens to abolish psychiatry's self-defined subject matter. (Boyle, 2011)

If you were repeatedly raped throughout your childhood, if you were terrified of the people who were supposed to be caring for you, if you had to get up and have breakfast with the people who'd hurt you the night before and pretend it hadn't happened, when you think about the mental contortions that some children have to use to survive with any sanity intact, how is it surprising that they develop ways of surviving, like cutting themselves or hearing voices? And psychiatrists have the audacity to talk about 'maladaptive coping'. What about adaptive coping? Why do we have to have the 'maladapting'? As I've said to psychiatrists, if you'd been subjected to the things I went through as a little girl, it's quite likely you would have used some of the same strategies. Why are you not saying, 'You're amazing! How did you survive these terrible things? Tell us more about this. We need to learn from you!' We should be championing these people who have survived these terrible experiences. We should be more curious about the methods they have used to survive. Where is our wonder that people have been subjected to horrific things are still here, still fighting for their lives? They're kind, they're funny, they're still here! Where is our celebration of that? Yet all we want to do is reduce them to a set of 'maladaptive coping strategies' and signs and symptoms of 'disorders'. How is it we still do this in 2019?

Another one is the stress-vulnerability hypothesis. Basically, it's a very simple pile of shit. What it's saying is that some of us are born with a genetic vulnerability to having mental health problems. I find that idea inherently offensive. What it's saying is, if I'd been a bit genetically stronger, a bit more genetically robust, somehow I would have survived better from the things that happened to me, which is a very insulting, hurtful assertion. And then I read this quote by the wonderful Mary Boyle and for me she perfectly sums up what is so problematic about this hypothesis. And it is a hypothesis that, like many things in psychiatry, is spoken of as if it were fact.

> The vulnerability-stress hypothesis… has proved to be an extraordinarily useful and effective mechanism for managing the potential threat to biological models… Its usefulness lies in its seeming reasonableness (who could deny that biological and psychological and social factors interact?) and its inclusiveness (it encompasses both the biological and the social – surely better than focusing on only one?), while at the same time it firmly maintains the primacy of biology… by making it look as if the 'stress' of the model consists of ordinary stresses which most of us would cope with, but which overwhelm only 'vulnerable' people. We are thus excused from examining too closely either the events themselves or their meaning to the 'vulnerable' person. (Boyle, 2002: 14)

We know from a huge amount of research what can lead to what are commonly diagnosed as 'severe mental illnesses'. And it's a long list (Read & Bentall, 2012):

- mother's ill health, poor nutrition and high stress during pregnancy
- being an unwanted pregnancy
- early loss of parents via death or abandonment
- attachment difficulties
- witnessing interparental violence
- intergenerational trauma
- dysfunctional parenting (particularly lack of affection and over-control)
- parental substance misuse, mental health problems and criminal behaviour
- childhood sexual, physical and emotional abuse
- childhood emotional or physical neglect
- bullying
- childhood medical illness
- war trauma
- poverty, racism and other forms of social inequality.

I'm now going to give you some examples of diagnoses from the new *DSM-5* (American Psychiatric Association, 2013).

Temper tantrums in children? Children who have more than three temper tantrums a month for a year are suffering from 'disruptive mood dysregulation disorder'.

Emotional reactions to the loss of a loved one that continue for more than two months? Still sad after two months? What's wrong with you? You've got 'major depressive disorder'.

Everyday forgetting, characteristic of old age? 'Minor neuro-cognitive disorder'.

And my personal favourite: *excessive eating more than 12 times in three months*. That's 'binge-eating disorder'.

They're funny, but they're not funny. Take 'disruptive mood dysregulation disorder' – what we know now is toddlers will be given very powerful psychotropic medications just when their very young brains are developing – that's what that diagnosis means. In fact, for all of these 'disorders', there will be an accompanying drug that some fucker is making a lot of money out of. That's what it boils down to.

This is darker and quite upsetting – from a paper by John Read and colleagues (2003) on hallucinations, delusions and 'thought disorder' in adult psychiatric inpatients with a history of childhood abuse. John Read went back through these patients' psychiatric notes and looked at how they had disclosed their experiences and how these experiences had been recorded.

For one, the records said:

> Sexual abuse: abused from an early age… Raped several times by strangers and violent partners… [believes] was being tortured by people getting into body, for example 'the Devil' and the 'Beast' and had bleeding secondary to inserting a bathroom hose into self, stating wanting to wash self as 'people are trying to put aliens into my body'.

Another, whose records reported childhood sexual and physical abuse and multiple rapes, was recorded as believing 'has never been a child but is an old man who had his penis gouged out and had silicone injected into chest and hips'. Another, whose chart documented childhood sexual abuse, also documented 'olfactory hallucinations (smells sperm)'. This is the bit that gets me – adding in brackets 'smells sperm'. I mean, what is going on there?

Here is another example, from one of the best-selling psychiatric textbooks in the country, about paintings by people with schizophrenia:

> Paintings by schizophrenia sufferers often have an odd, eerie quality. In many cases the usual artistic conventions are disregarded, and the pictures include written comments, digits and other idiosyncratic material. For example, Guardian Angels was painted by Else B, an institutionalized schizophrenic. In all her works, the legs of angels are painted as though they had fused at the top, to make sure that 'nothing happens there'. (Prinzhorn, 1972)

I mean, hello? Would anyone else looking at that picture at least wonder if Else had experienced some kind of sexual violation? We can't know but I might want to explore that with her if it felt appropriate. But no, this is weird, idiosyncratic shit; this is 'schizophrenic'.

Returning to language, Mary Boyle has also researched how the language of vulnerability locates the blame and responsibility elsewhere (2003). She tabulated the ways in which the 'language of vulnerability' is used to 'divert attention from oppression'. So, for example, a statement that 'Old people are vulnerable to hypothermia' actually means 'The government doesn't pay a high enough state pension for older people to pay their heating bills'; and 'Unassertive people are vulnerable to being bullied at work' translates into 'Managers in some workplaces pick on weaker employees'.

And we come back to this question of psychiatric terminology. I think terms like hallucinations, delusions, thought disorder, personality disorder, schizophrenia, bipolar… all of this jargon enables an apparent clinical assessment that creates an illusion –I would go as far as to say delusion – of neutral objectivity. To quote Sami Timimi (2005), a member of the Critical Psychiatry Network, diagnosis is 'subjective opinion masquerading as fact'. There's no blood test, no brain scan – basically, it's my opinion against yours.

It's actually subjective opinion about someone's subjective experience, masquerading as a fact. Because if you are in a position of power and you are in a setting where this kind of discourse is acceptable, then it gets adopted.

Doublethink invalidates; it mystifies; it renders unintelligible normal reactions to abnormal circumstances. It facilitates decontextualising, diminishment, distancing and denial of devastating experiences. What it results in is collusion and complicity because it focuses on the deficits of individuals rather than the assaults of the perpetrators. Where is the curiosity about all the people who are perpetrating these crimes? We only label people who have suffered at the hands of the perpetrators of injustices.

For me, as someone who was sexually abused as a child, it's very clear who my perpetrators were, but politically, they can be at a number of different levels. Mary Boyle again:

> … child abuse and neglect, school and workplace bullying, domestic and sexual violence, discrimination, poverty and unemployment… events [which] involve relatively powerful groups – governments, corporations, men, white people, adults – damaging less powerful groups. In the case of emotional distress, then, context seems to include or even equate to the operation of power. (Boyle, 2011)

This is ultimately what we are talking about – the operation of power. And I want to ram this point home because I am very proud to be part of the working group that came up with the Power Threat Meaning Framework (Johnstone & Boyle, 2018) that locates power as central to all mental health crises in some shape or form, and that is bang on the nail.

'Diagnosing' someone with 'schizophrenia' is one of the most damaging
things one human being can do to another. Re-defining someone's reality
for them is the most insidious and the most devastating form of power we
can use. (Johnstone, 2013)

In fact, you can probably replace 'schizophrenia' with any number of diagnoses. To say to me, when I'm disclosing what these people did to me, 'These things didn't actually happen. You're psychotic and you're having false memories,' is as big an abuse of power as any. When the people in our society who are meant to protect you, who are meant to offer you solace and comfort when you've been really damaged as a small child, reiterate the same words and blame you for it, wow…

What the research is saying (Read, Bentall & Fosse, 2009) is that there are many reasons why people end up having serious breakdowns, including inequality. There's tons of research that shows that when you live in a society where there's a greater disparity in incomes between rich and poor there's more mental illness in the general population. Apparently the most wealthy, well developed nation in the world, America, has the highest rates of people with a diagnosis of 'mental illness'. And if you look at the statistics for people who have been sexually abused in childhood, you'll find that, if you've endured three kinds of abuse – sexual and physical abuse and bullying for example – you are 18 times more likely to experience 'psychosis', and if you've experienced five types, it increases your chances about 193 times (Shevlin, Dorahy & Adamson, 2007).

There's another piece of research that shows if you have 'psychosis' you are three times more likely to have experienced childhood sexual abuse than if you have another diagnosis, and 15 times more likely to have been abused than people who haven't been diagnosed with a 'mental illness' at all (Bebbington et al, 2004). In research terms, those are mind-blowing statistics. We are talking about a dose effect. It's blindingly obvious. Then they show you slides that show how bits of the brain have closed down in people with a 'schizophrenia' diagnosis, but what they don't show are slides showing what happens to the brain when you've been sexually abused as a child. Trauma is what causes changes in people's brains – trauma, abuse, adversity. This is what we need to remember:

The knowledge of horrible events periodically intrudes into public awareness
but it is rarely retained for long. Denial, repression and dissociation operate on
a social as well as an individual level. (Herman, 1992)

The take-home message is we have a big battle on our hands. We've got a massive system that doesn't just prop up the medical system, it keeps our society the way it is. The people who are the most hurt in our society, who are the most oppressed and have experienced the worst things, are the people who are going to be subjected to the greatest coercion in psychiatry. This is how we treat people who have suffered the most already.

What's to be done?

I get despairing about mental health sometimes. Sometimes it just feels like nothing's changing. I went out for dinner with my friend John Read the other day, and I said, 'What's different? Has anything changed?' And he said, 'Jacqui, we have done all the research. We know what drives people mad. What we need to do now is just stop doing it.' But that would take a radical shift in our society.

So, what is to be done? First, don't give up. I've been working for years trying to change services and I feel pretty depressed sometimes about how much progress we have made. But if you are a professional working in mental health services, one of the things you can do is to refuse to be colonised by the biomedical model. Don't adopt this pseudo-scientific language just to fit in.

Rebecca Solnit, author and environmental and human rights campaigner, writes that work around human rights often starts by 'reframing the status quo as an outrage'. She says (2012): 'Change the language and you've begun to change the reality or at least to open the status quo to question.'

So, decolonise the medicalised language of human experience. Don't use phrases like 'auditory hallucinations'; use ordinary, non pathologising language like 'hearing voices'.

Reframe and reclaim ordinary language that restores meaning and context and is firmly rooted in people's lived, subjective experiences. So, when psychiatrists say, 'This is person is non-compliant,' say: 'This person has her own ideas about what she wants to do.'

There's a whole list of other things you can do in your daily practice to subvert the status quo:

- deconstruct the biomedical model and the traditional relationship of dominant, expert clinician and passive, recipient patient
- share power – advocate and practice mutually respectful collaborations between experts by experience and experts by profession
- take a stand – have the courage to bear witness to and name taboos, injustices, outrages
- stop using scientifically meaningless, stigmatising words that focus on deficit and chronicity, like 'schizophrenia' and medicalising terms like 'mental illness'
- reframe and reclaim ordinary language that restores meaning and context and is firmly rooted in people's lived, subjective experiences
- ensure service users are involved in the management of, and training about, mental health services
- ask service users about their past and how they think that relates to their current problems – reject the 'can of worms' fallacy
- help your colleagues focus on recovery not pathology.

And form alliances. We can't do this on our own. Form alliances between progressive professional organisations and groups of service users and family groups.

And if you are a person who has to use services and their diagnoses for whatever reason – because you need the support, you need the welfare benefits, you need the passport of diagnosis to open certain doors – fine, but don't buy their version of your reality.

Don't buy the bullshit.
Know your own truth.
Define your own reality.
Do not let anyone else define your reality for you.

References

American Psychiatric Association (2013). *Diagnostic and Statistical Manual of Mental Disorders* (5th ed). Washington, DC: American Psychiatric Association.

American Psychiatric Association (1994). *Diagnostic and Statistical Manual of Mental Disorders* (4th ed). Washington, DC: American Psychiatric Association.

Bebbington PE, Bhugra D, Brugha T, Singleton N, Farrell M, Jenkins R et al (2004). Psychosis, victimisation and childhood disadvantage: evidence from the second British National Survey of Psychiatric Morbidity. *British Journal of Psychiatry 185*: 220–226.

Bowlby J (1988). *A Secure Base: clinical applications of attachment theory.* London: Routledge.

Boyle M (2011). Making the world go away and how psychiatry and psychology benefits. In: Rapley M, Moncrieff J, Dillon J. *De-Medicalizing Misery: psychiatry, psychology and the human condition.* Basingstoke: Palgrave Macmillan (pp27–43).

Boyle M (2003). The dangers of vulnerability. *Clinical Psychology 24*: 27–30.

Boyle M (2002). It's all done with smoke and mirrors. Or, how to create the illusion of a schizophrenic brain disease. *Clinical Psychology 12*: 9–16.

Einstein A (1941/1942). The common language of science. Presentation to the British Association for the Advancement of Science. *Advancement of Science 2*(5).

Herman J (1992). *Trauma and Recovery: the aftermath of violence – from domestic abuse to political terror.* New York, NY: Basic Books.

Johnstone L (2013). Time to abolish psychiatric diagnosis? [Blog.] *Mad in America*; 1 January. www.madinamerica.com/2013/01/time-to-abolish-psychiatric-diagnosis/ (accessed 15 June 2019).

Johnstone L, Boyle M with Cromby J, Dillon J, Harper D, Kinderman P, Longden E, Pilgrim D, Read J (2018). *The Power Threat Meaning Framework: towards the identification of patterns in emotional distress, unusual experiences and troubled or troubling behaviour, as an alternative to functional psychiatric diagnosis.* Leicester: British Psychological Society.

McArthur T (ed) (1992). *The Oxford Companion to the English Language.* Oxford: Oxford University Press (p321).

Orwell G (1949). *Nineteen Eighty-Four.* London: Secker & Warburg.

Prinzhorn H (1972). *Artistry of the Mentally Ill* (von Brockdorff E, trans). New York, NY: Springer Science & Business Media.

Read J, Agar K, Argyle N, Aderhold V (2003). Sexual and physical abuse during childhood and adulthood as predictors of hallucinations, delusions and thought disorder. *Psychology and Psychotherapy: Theory, Research and Practice 76*(1): 1–22.

Read J, Bentall RP (2012). Editorial: Negative childhood experiences and mental health: theoretical, clinical and primary prevention implications. *British Journal of Psychiatry 200*: 89–91.

Read J, Bentall RP, Fosse R (2009). Time to abandon the bio-bio-bio model of psychosis: exploring the epigenetic and psychological mechanisms by which adverse life events lead to psychotic symptoms. *Epidemiologia e Psichiatria Sociale 18*: 299–310.

Romme M, Escher S, Dillon J, Corstens D, Morris M (2009). *Living with Voices: 50 stories of recovery.* Ross-on-Wye: PCCS Books.

Santayana G (2016). *The Life of Reason: the phases of human progress (1905-1906). Vol I: Reason in common sense.* Victoria: Leopold Classic Library.

Shevlin M, Dorahy MJ, Adamson G (2007). Trauma and psychosis: an analysis of the National Comorbidity Survey. *American Journal of Psychiatry 164*(1):166–169.

Solnit R (2012). Words are the greatest weapon for political activists. [Blog.] *The Guardian*; 29 October. www.theguardian.com/commentisfree/2012/oct/29/words-greatest-weapon-political-activists (accessed 15 June 2019).

Timimi S (2005). *Naughty Boys: antisocial behaviour, ADHD and the role of culture.* Basingstoke: Palgrave Macmillan.

20 | There's an intruder in our house! Counselling, psychotherapy and the biomedical model of emotional distress

Jo Watson

I've been a psychotherapist for 24 years, but I think my days in this profession are numbered. The truth is, I'm not sure how long I can continue to align myself with a profession that, despite all its talk of person-centred, humanistic values, seems happy to share its house with the biomedical model of psychiatry.

The counselling profession (and in that I include psychotherapy) is helping to endorse a medical understanding of emotional distress that is based on 'What is wrong with you?' and not 'What has happened to you?' (Felitti et al, 1998). In short, counselling and psychotherapy are serving to support the psychiatric propaganda challenged in every chapter of this book.

It wasn't always like this. In the early 1990s, I joined a profession that held a shared belief about the nature of human emotional distress. We understood that the many forms of human suffering we witnessed – ranging from feeling low and suicidal to self-injury, hearing voices, overwhelming anxiety and dissociative experiences – were responses and reactions to what had happened in people's lives and, in many cases, the resourceful and creative coping strategies they had developed in order to survive. I and my fellow therapists clearly and consistently made links between emotional distress and causal factors like poverty, racism and abuse. There was a deep, collective 'knowing' that social circumstances were linked directly to human suffering and this acknowledgement translated into a connection with the political arena, which for me was a crucial part of the whole picture.

Yet, as I write this, almost two and a half decades later, I can hardly recognise that profession. The precious, collective 'good stuff' that drew so many of us to this work has been consumed by a biomedical monster that has crept into our house and made itself very much at home. In fact, I don't feel this is my home anymore – and nor, I suspect, do thousands like me.

Let me give you some examples of what I mean.

In the late 1980s, while at college, I was involved with numerous women's survivor groups; in the early 1990s, before embarking on my psychotherapy training, I was working with young women survivors in a residential setting in Birmingham. In both contexts, over an eight-year period, despite the extraordinary amount of emotional distress I encountered, there was very little mention of psychiatric diagnoses. By 1996, I'd qualified and taken up my first therapeutic post at Sandwell Rape and Sexual Abuse Centre. Here I saw up to 15 girls and young women a week and worked with many more over the phone or in therapeutic groups. In the next seven years, I only came across a very small handful of survivors who had been given a psychiatric diagnosis. Back then, I took it for granted that we lived in a culture that, despite its many problems, did by and large acknowledge that emotional distress was caused by what had happened to a person, rather than by a biological illness. The Labour government of the day poured funding into community support and services to address particular social issues. Rape Crisis services had never been so financially secure.

It could be argued that this contributed to an unhelpful 'professionalisation' of counselling, as well as the inevitable political compromises that organisations had to make in order to secure that valuable government funding. (That's another book!) Still, the voluntary/third sector grew rapidly and important links were being made between social issues and emotional distress.

My seven years at Rape Crisis were also supported by a feminist philosophy that made direct links between the power structures in society and sexual violence. Indeed, the whole wider women's movement was giving out a clear non-pathologising message to survivors: 'Your distress is a result of what happened to you and it is an appropriate response/reaction. It is not your fault.'

I had no idea, back then in the mid-90s, that several years down the line we would be seeing so many people coming to us either with a psychiatric diagnosis or seeking a diagnostic explanation of their problems. We are seeing survivors of abuse typically labelled with 'borderline personality disorder', children labelled with 'attention deficit hyperactivity disorder'. To quote the title of the events I now organise, there seems to be a 'disorder' for everyone and for everything. As James Davies points out in Chapter 6 of this book, in the last 35 years the DSM has 'more than doubled the number of mental disorders believed to exist'. He goes on to point out that the lowering of diagnostic thresholds has resulted in more people being diagnosed with a psychiatric disorder than ever before.

Indeed, the biomedical model of emotional distress has woven itself, perhaps inextricably, into the very fabric of society. These days, we routinely use the language of illness and disorder to explain human emotional distress. These messages of illness come at us, as propaganda does, from all directions: media, politics, education and entertainment such as soap operas, film and music. National treasures – football heroes, actors, musicians, media celebrities – have all played their part – albeit with the best of intentions. Comedians Ruby Wax and Stephen Fry have both climbed on board the biomedical bandwagon while attempting to combat the stigma surrounding 'depression' and 'bipolar disorder'.

Wax launched her career as the 'poster girl for mental health' with *Losing It*, first staged in London in 2010. I was in the audience at the pilot for this show and was shocked to witness what I can only describe as a festival of pathology. Wax told us that mental 'illness' is the same as physical illness. She compared 'depression' to diabetes; she explained that some brains were 'broken' and that medication 'managed' the brokenness. The show was loaded from beginning to end with medicalised language – words and phrases like 'disease', 'genes', 'severe, lifelong conditions', 'chemical imbalance', 'symptoms', 'treatment' – I could go on; no links were drawn between trauma and adversity and emotional distress. For Wax, 'depression is an illness', not an understandable response to life's adversities.

Since then Wax has continued to spread the biomedical message of 'mental illness' and is now an ambassador for Mind, one of the UK's leading UK mental health charities, as well President of the relationship counselling organisation Relate.

The equally influential and well-loved actor Stephen Fry (currently President of Mind) similarly uses his celebrity profile and personal story to perpetuate biomedical myths about emotional distress. As their titles suggest, his 2007 BBC series *The Secret Life of the Manic Depressive* and his 2017 follow-up BBC film *The Not So Secret Life of the Manic Depressive: 10 Years On* both presented a very medicalised view of emotional distress that, like Ruby Wax's show, made no attempt to link distress with life experiences. Professor Richard Bentall, a leading psychologist and researcher, was prompted by Fry's media utterances to write an open letter to him to challenge his consistent failure to discuss the non-biological causes of mental distress and the impact of his message on people with this diagnosis:

> … many psychiatric patients in Britain feel that services too often ignore their life stories, treating them more like surgical or neurological patients than people whose difficulties have arisen in response to challenging circumstances. To make matters worse, research shows that exclusively biological theories of mental illness contribute to the stigma experienced by mental health patients, which I know you want to reduce… The biomedical model of mental illness, which your programme showcased, makes it all too easy to believe that humans belong to two sub-species: the mentally well and the mentally ill. (Bentall, 2016)

All of these media-driven messages translate unsurprisingly into more and more people understanding their distress and suffering in diagnostic terms, whether or not they have been given an official label or not. People think of themselves as having 'anxiety disorder', 'depression', 'bipolar disorder' and so on, and attribute their 'illness' to 'biochemical imbalances' or genetic factors. Many have internalised these labels into their identity, along with the belief that these are 'lifelong conditions' that can only be managed with psychotropic drugs.

Others have accepted the message that overwhelming anxiety and desperate sadness can come out of nowhere and be totally unrelated to what is currently happening or has happened in their lives. The language of 'diagnosis and disorder' has replaced the everyday language we once used to describe emotional states, and the acronyms of psychiatry are now part of our everyday conversations.

What does this mean for counsellors, psychotherapists and our clients?

This question recently came up on the Drop the Disorder! Facebook group[1] – a forum where people can discuss these ideas and challenge the culture of psychiatric diagnosis. Orla McLoughlin, a student counsellor based in Dublin, explained that, in her work as a counsellor in a college/university setting, many of her student clients were coming to counselling with a medicalised understanding of their problems. She said that, in her experience, clients were 'increasingly entrenched in the illness model' and that it was very common for a person to talk about 'symptoms' that were, for them, seemingly unrelated to anything else going on in their lives. 'They may say that the reason they feel the way they do is because they "have anxiety" and need coping strategies.' For Orla, this was unsurprising as the message that emotional distress is indicative of something being medically wrong rather than being connected to experience is a strong one: 'It's just the dominant narrative on campus about "mental illness" where very little link is made between mental distress and personal experience.'

Orla's comments certainly echo my own experience in my counselling work, especially in recent years. Whether they have an official diagnosis or not, many people are coming to therapy with a belief that their difficulties stem from one disorder or another and consequently understand their emotional distress in a medicalised way.

Many counsellors and psychotherapists would, and indeed do say that it is the role and responsibility of a counsellor /psychotherapist to work with a client's own understanding of their situation. This is usually true, but I would argue that, if a client understands themselves as having life-long, life-limiting illness, with no evidence that this is so, it is our ethical responsibility as counsellors to challenge that, appropriately and sensitively.

I will use an anonymised example of some work I did with a client, who I shall call Yasmin, to discuss this. Yasmin came to therapy at the recommendation of her GP who had prescribed antidepressants for what he had called 'clinical

---

1. www.adisorder4everyone.com/new-facebook-group/ (accessed 15 June 2019).

depression'. This was the reason she gave for embarking on therapy: 'I have clinical depression and my GP says that counselling may help.' When I asked what she wanted to get from counselling, she said that she wanted to learn how to come to terms with her condition and to find ways of coping when she was particularly low. Yasmin believed that something was wrong with her brain chemistry that meant that these bouts of severe 'depression' would be a life-long reality for her.

Should I have accepted Yasmin's 'chemical imbalance' belief and facilitated a process that helped her to find her peace with this? To me, this would have meant my using my professional authority to collude with what is at best a highly disputed premise and at worst an extremely dangerous falsehood.

Instead, I gently explored Yasmin's own goals for the therapy through careful, respectful questions to find out how *she* understood the diagnosis of 'clinical depression' as well as where this understanding came from and what it meant to her. Yasmin had never thought about this before and, as a result of simply being asked those questions, began a gradual process of making her own sense of what was going on for her.

She told me that her GP's diagnosis of 'clinical depression' had emerged from a 10-minute consultation and that his explanation had been affirmed for her by information she'd gathered online as a result of googling 'clinical depression'.

I shared my belief that every person has the right to make their own choices about how they understand the distress they experience, and that there are other ways of understanding the distress she was experiencing, if she wanted to explore them. We then left the subject there, to come back to if she ever wanted.

As our therapeutic relationship progressed, however, Yasmin started to open up about painful experiences she'd had experienced in early adulthood and began to remember how these experiences had impacted emotionally back then and how she'd had to bury her feelings because it wasn't safe to feel them in the violent situation she had been in. She had never been in a place where it was safe to feel and express those feelings and so had pushed the story that accompanied them so far away it was almost forgotten. 'Clinical depression' had become Yasmin's story, but it was not her truth. That had been obscured underneath the label and very nearly lost forever.

Yasmin's counselling journey was an intensely painful process but it enabled her to make sense of the 'depression' she had been experiencing for many years. After some time, she came to reject the diagnosis 'clinical depression' and, with the support of her GP, gradually tapered off the drugs that had been prescribed.

Of course, Yasmin's situation is not representative of *all* clients who come to therapy with firm beliefs about a mental health disorder or condition. I have worked with plenty of people over the years who have chosen to stick with a diagnostic understanding and I could understand and respect why in all of those cases. However, I always *presented the option* to explore a different understanding. To have colluded with the 'mental illness' narrative by affirming that I accepted it would have been both dishonest and unethical. Ultimately, we do not have to share our clients' opinions and beliefs, but we do have to accept that sometimes our clients make choices that we wouldn't.

While Yasmin may not be representative of *all* clients who come to therapy with a medicalised understanding of their distress, she is, in my experience, representative of the majority when it comes to her willingness and openness to explore how emotional distress is understood. If, as a therapist, I had accepted without any further explanation her initial objective of 'coming to terms' with what she had understood as a 'life-long illness', I'm sure that the process and outcome of our work together would have been dramatically different – as, indeed, would have been her life going forward.

This is because psychiatric diagnosis inevitably steers people away from making the connections between adverse life events and experiences and the understandable distress they suffer as a result. This leaves the painful parts of people's lives – parts that desperately need to be acknowledged, validated and made sense of – effectively ignored and unresolved.

How does this fit with the objectives of counselling?

However, this is not the only reason we should be concerned with psychiatric diagnosis. It also offers a convenient scapegoat for governments and our political representatives. As long as individual illness is accepted as being the primary cause of distress, the real causes go unnamed, and those responsible for them are effectively let off the hook. Richard Bentall's letter clearly states this, and others have reported it elsewhere (see, notably, Wilkinson & Pickett, 2010, 2018; also, for example, Read, Bentall & Fosse, 2009): statistically, the second strongest predictor of emotional distress is poverty, and the first is relative poverty and social inequality.

By colluding with the diagnostic model, counselling and psychotherapy are not only failing to hear the stories of the individuals we work with; we are also colluding with state-sanctioned power structures that serve to perpetuate the very factors that are bringing clients to our counselling rooms. How is that ethical?

Denial and collusion

As the chapters by James Davies, Lucy Johnstone and others in this book make clear, the diagnoses that end up in the American Psychiatric Association's *Diagnostic and Statistical Manual of Mental Disorders* (APA, 2013) and its equivalent, the World Health Organization's *International Classification of Diseases* (WHO, 2018), are subjective opinions with no scientific basis, voted through by committees of psychiatrists. The initial, detailed revelations of the unscientific nature of psychiatric diagnoses are also detailed in the introduction to this book.

Given that we know the scientific validity of psychiatric diagnosis to be highly disputed, coupled with the fact that it conflicts with the fundamental theoretical underpinnings of counselling and psychotherapy, it is very difficult to understand why therapists are not protesting in large numbers about it. Instead, the opposite is true. Many counsellors and psychotherapists simply don't accept the relevance of the debate. The following quote was directed at me in a discussion on a counsellors' Facebook group in 2018, and it nicely exemplifies this position:

> The debate around psychiatric diagnosis is not relevant to counselling and psychotherapy. We don't think in those terms, it's not our thing.

It is certainly true that most counselling theory is not compatible with psychiatric diagnosis. Person-centred theory is an obvious example, with its emphasis on regarding the client as the expert on their own experience and director of their own healing. Rogers himself was vehemently opposed to psychiatric diagnosis. Pete Sanders, person-centred counsellor and writer, has always been puzzled as to why counsellors 'abdicated the radical position occupied by client-centred therapy in the 1950s to become tacit supporters of the medical psychiatric system?' (Sanders, 2017). Yet the fundamental principles of non-judgemental, unconditional positive regard and the belief in human beings' capacity to achieve our best potential, given the right circumstances, seem to have become dislodged by diagnostic thinking.

I strongly disagree with the counsellor who suggested that psychiatric diagnosis isn't an issue for counsellors. I will now offer examples that support my case.

1. Allegiances with medical model groups and organisations

Most of our professional organisations support the mainstream mental health charities and organisations, such as Mind, Sane, Bipolar UK, Rethink, Time to Change and the Mental Health Foundation, on social media. These organisations promote the medical-model, 'illness like any other' viewpoint in their anti-stigma messages. They talk about 'severe life-long mental illness' (Bipolar UK, undated), and people being born with 'obsessive compulsive disorder'; in 2017, the anti-stigma campaigning organisation Time to Change ran a campaign with the subtitle 'I was born with OCD and it's part of me' (Time to Change, 2017).

One might argue that retweeting and liking the tweets of such organisations is no big deal, but it tells the rest of the world where we as a profession are coming from and what we understand about mental distress.

We don't think in those terms, it's not our thing.

2. Core training

Many psychotherapy courses now have compulsory mental health components, some of which include placements in psychiatric services. Students are asked to differentiate clients into diagnostic categories in case studies and in supervision groups, on the basis of their 'presenting symptoms'. Tutors and trainees routinely talk about clients with 'mental illnesses'. Psychiatric diagnosis is being taught uncritically on many courses and the *DSM* features on course reading lists up and down the country.

We don't think in those terms, it's not our thing.

3. Advertising counselling and psychotherapy services

The online Counselling Directory (www.counselling-directory.org.uk) is the largest such directory in the UK for private therapists to advertise their services. It requires its subscribers to tick boxes to indicate the 'issues' they work with. Many of the boxes are titled with *DSM* diagnoses, including 10 that list different types of 'personality disorder':

Antisocial personality disorder
Avoidant personality disorder
Borderline personality disorder
Dependent personality disorder
Histrionic personality disorder
Narcissistic personality disorder
Obsessive compulsive personality disorder
Paranoid personality disorder
Schizoid personality disorder
Schizotypal personality disorder

We don't think in those terms, it's not our thing.

4. Use of medicalised language and diagnostic terms

Counsellors and psychotherapists are routinely using the language of diagnosis and disorder and *DSM* terminology, including the acronyms of psychiatric diagnosis, without a second thought, as though it has always been our native tongue. It hasn't.

Here are just a few examples of phrases that I've seen used on counselling Facebook groups, which have been accepted without any meaningful challenge:

It sounds like she's a schizophrenic.

I suggest you google dissociative identity disorder – it's obviously that.

Be careful working with borderline clients if you have no specific training or experience of working with them.

That's sounds like a narcissistic personality disorder to me.

I'm pretty sure my client has oppositional defiant disorder.

As Jacqui Dillon and other contributors to this book have argued, language matters.

We don't think in those terms, it's not our thing.

5. Continuing professional development

There is a vibrant and thriving market in continuing professional development (CPD) for counsellors and psychotherapists. Indeed, it is a formal requirement for registration with most professional bodies. A quick glance at the websites and pages of most counselling publications shows how deeply embedded the narrative of psychiatric diagnosis is within the courses on offer. Training organisations offer certificates in 'Working with Borderlines', 'Working with OCD', and 'Working with Dissociative Identity Disorder', to name just a few that I've spotted in a random trawl. Many counsellors believe that they need this extra training to be able to work ethically with people who have been given a particular psychiatric diagnosis. This is unsurprising when their own professional bodies are both advertising and running such courses, but it is also deeply disturbing.

We don't think in those terms, it's not our thing.

6. The future of the counselling profession

As I write this (June 2019), the three largest organisations representing counselling and psychotherapy have come together in an unprecedented joint endeavour to map out the so-called competencies of their respective members. The United Kingdom Council for Psychotherapy (UKCP), the British Association for Counselling and Psychotherapy (BACP) and the British Psychoanalytic Council (BPC) between them represent some 60,000 practitioners – the bulk of practitioners in the UK – and their aim is to map out the level of skills at which these members can practise on completion of their initial training. This project, the Scope of Practice and Education for the Counselling and Psychotherapy Professions (SCoPEd), aims to agree a 'shared, evidence-based generic competence framework to inform the training requirements, competences and practice standards for counsellors and psychotherapists working with adults' (BACP, 2018). The framework will identify 'the knowledge, skills and values that are relevant to counselling and psychotherapy', and essentially delineate at what level of skill each member can practise.

The initial consultation provoked a furore of negative response on social media. Much of the criticism was around the encroaching professionalisation of counselling, and what is perceived as a move to make counselling a higher-level profession and able to compete on a level NHS mental health playing field with psychology and, even, psychiatry. But there was also vehement criticism of the language used to describe the varied competences, particularly at the 'higher' level of qualification and practice. For example, competences for psychotherapists and 'advanced qualified counsellors' include (BACP/BCP/UKCP, 2018):

> 2.4.a Ability to critically appraise the nature of 'psychopathological' and 'normal' functioning and distinguish between them, during assessment and throughout therapy (advanced qualified counsellor)
> 2.5.a Ability to recognise more significant mental health symptoms and difficulties, and know when and how to refer on (advanced qualified counsellor)
> 2.4.b Ability to understand medical diagnosis of mental disorders and the impact of psychotropic medication during assessment and throughout therapy (psychotherapist)

Even the 'qualified counsellor' can 'draw upon knowledge of common mental health problems and their presentation during assessment and throughout therapy' (2.4). One BACP member blogged:

> This is about more than language. This isn't just a few misplaced words. The entire thrust of the research is about differentiating counselling from psychotherapy, and enshrining diagnostic-leaning trainings in the process. (Stevens, 2019)

The inference is very clear – working with diagnosis is indicative of professional status and superiority. Such an ambition for our profession not only takes us in the completely wrong direction as far as the pathologising of distress is concerned; if this consultative framework is enshrined as an accepted definition of competency, it will dictate all future training and standards of professional practice and inevitably drag us deeper down the biomedical model rabbit hole.

We don't think in those terms, it's not our thing.

To me, these six points summarise the clear messages we as a profession are giving out to the public and to policy-makers about what counsellors and psychotherapists do and what we believe in. We are also sending the same messages to new counsellors and psychotherapists who represent the future of the profession and, perhaps most concerning of all, we are absorbing these messages ourselves and passing them on to the people we work with.

Why do we collude?

The justification for this ongoing collusion seems to stem, at least in part, from the belief that, if a client already understands their problems in this way, we must respect and work with that understanding. But there are also many people who think that there is no real harm in using or promoting it. However, as clinical psychologist Lucy Johnstone (2016) has pointed out, it is very rare for someone treated in our mental health services to be given a choice about whether they want a psychiatric diagnosis. Furthermore, any ongoing support from our public health and social care services and welfare benefits system is usually conditional on having such a label. It makes sense that people would perceive diagnosis, at least initially, as bringing benefits and as a welcome relief because, on some levels, it validates their distress in a still heavily stigmatising world and opens doors to support.

Our professional associations argue that they need to 'occupy an important middle ground' on the issue of diagnosis, as stated by a senior executive officer within BACP (Jackson, 2019). But, when it comes to psychiatric diagnosis, I think this 'balanced' position is very problematic. We rightly refuse to accept racist and homophobic terms. The same should apply to pathologising terminology. We can promote open discussion without colluding with the premise that psychiatric diagnoses are legitimate, scientifically valid and reliable categories. Furthermore, is this position ethical once we understand that the diagnostic model is rarely freely chosen and has such far-reaching damaging consequences?

Lucy Johnstone is among a growing number of experts who consider it to be an ethical responsibility for therapists to not collude with the concept of diagnosis: 'It can no longer be considered professionally, scientifically or ethically justifiable to present psychiatric diagnoses as if they were valid statements about people and their difficulties' (Johnstone & Boyle, 2018: 85).

I would argue that, by accepting the story of diagnosis without question, we are curtailing the counselling/psychotherapeutic process; we are closing down the exploration of people's stories, which we know is a central part of the therapeutic process. Many stories are going unheard, unacknowledged and inevitably lost forever because, once a psychiatric diagnosis has been accepted as the explanation for the distress, no other explanation is needed or sought. The 'illness' becomes the story.

Judith Herman, in her book *Trauma and Recovery* (1992), talks about how healing is achieved precisely through the telling of one's story. She talks about the 'restorative power of truth telling' with a safe witness and ally. This processing and reconstruction of trauma memories is key to healing, she argues:

> In the second stage of recovery the survivor tells the story of the trauma. She tells it completely, in depth and in detail. This work of reconstruction actually transforms the traumatic memory so that it can be integrated into the survivor's life story. (Herman, 1992: 175)

Survivor and activist Beth Filson (2016: 22) sums this up perfectly for me:

> Until we are able to use our own words to tell our own stories, the context we find ourselves in – in this case, the psychiatric system – says our stories for us, and usually gets it wrong. In the context of the medical model, the story we learn to say is that we are ill. We begin to see ourselves as ill. We tell stories of illness, and the psychiatric system, and, by extension, society accepts illness as the story of our distress. Being able to tell your own story – not the illness story – sets a new social context: one in which mad people are seen in a new light.

In part, she concludes, 'healing happens in the re-storying of our lives' (2016: 23).

So what do we do about it?

I believe that, at the very least, the counselling and psychotherapy professional bodies should be offering some basic guidance on psychiatric diagnosis. Professional bodies have a responsibility to offer accurate information on this issue so that therapists can be in a better position to facilitate informed choice for clients.

People can and, of course, should make up their own minds about how they best understand their distress but, as is the case with prescribed drugs, informed decisions can only be made when people have access to all the relevant information on which to base their decision.

How do we work with diagnostic assumptions in the therapy room? To summarise what I wrote about my work with Yasmin, challenging diagnosis in the counselling room needs to be done slowly, carefully and within a trusting relationship. We need to gently invite exploration that may help a client to make their own links and connections. We need to be witnesses to stories that may, up until this point, have been unheard and uninvited, and to make links to social factors and the wider context that these stories are inevitably part of. Above all, I think we should strive towards bringing our full selves to the work and allow our own stories and experience of being human to consciously inform it. We should work with honesty and integrity and be equipped with evidence-based information to ensure that we do not collude unknowingly with the misinformation that surrounds us all.

I would add that this means not being afraid to recommend resources if a person wishes to explore the issue of psychiatric diagnosis further. Suggest books and websites that give people access to the discussions and debates about the validity of diagnosis and its advantages and disadvantages. Information is crucial if people are to be empowered to make up their own minds.

And, at the risk of sounding nostalgic, we could all do with reminding ourselves of some of the fundamental principles and values of counselling and psychotherapy:

- the capacity of the individual to achieve their potential
- the refusal to collude with oppressive 'norms'
- the links between emotional distress and the wider social context
- the commitment to hear a person's story
- the centrality of a trusted relationship in which a person can safely and authentically connect with the truth of their lives.

None of this is new.

My hope is that those counsellors and psychotherapists who are presently denying there is problem and those who are colluding with it will realise that diagnostic explanations have no place in our profession; that they have no scientific basis and are actively anti-therapeutic in that they serve to shut down people's stories and prevent authentic exploration and sharing of experiences, which are such a core part of healing.

My hope is that we, the counselling and psychotherapy profession, will revisit our own story, its roots and its values, and confront the incongruity between them and the current trend in our practice. We will then embark on a radical process of reclaiming our core values and our original non-pathologising language and join our psychology colleagues in taking a stand against the pseudo-science of psychiatric diagnosis that contradicts its very identity.

In short, my optimistic future would see counselling and psychotherapy telling the unwelcome intruder to leave our house. There is no place for it here.

References

American Psychiatric Association (1994). *Diagnostic and Statistical Manual of Mental Disorders* (4th ed). Washington, DC: American Psychiatric Association.

American Psychiatric Association (1980). *Diagnostic and Statistical Manual of Mental Disorders* (3rd ed). Washington, DC: American Psychiatric Association.

BACP (2018). *FAQs about ScoPEd.* [Online.] BACP. www.bacp.co.uk/about-us/advancing-the-profession/scoped/scoped-faqs/ (accessed 29 June 2019).

BACP/BCP/UKCP (2018). *SCoPEd: a draft framework for the practice and education of counselling and psychotherapy.* Lutterworth/London: BACP/BPC/UKCP. www.bacp.co.uk/media/5161/scoped-competency-framework.pdf (accessed 29 June 2019).

Bentall R (2016). *All in the brain?* [Blog.] Canterbury Christchurch University; 19 February. https://blogs.canterbury.ac.uk/discursive/all-in-the-brain/ (accessed 13 June 2019).

Bipolar UK (undated) *Could mood swings mean bipolar?* [Online.] Bipolar UK. www.bipolaruk.org/FAQs/leaflet-could-mood-swings-mean-bipolar (accessed 31 July 2019).

Felitti V, Anda R, Nordenberg D, Williamson DF, Spitz AM, Edwards V Koss MP, Marks JS (1998). Relationship of childhood abuse and household dysfunction to many of the leading causes of death in adults: the Adverse Childhood Experiences (ACE) study. *American Journal of Preventive Medicine* 14(4): 245–258.

Filson B (2016). The haunting can end: trauma-informed approaches in healing from abuse and adversity. In: Russo J, Sweeney A (eds). *Searching for a Rose Garden*. Monmouth: PCCS Books (pp20–24).

Herman J (1992). *Trauma and Recovery: the aftermath of violence – from domestic abuse to political terror*. New York, NY: Basic Books.

Jackson C (2019). Who needs a diagnosis? *Therapy Today 30*(1): 8–11.

Johnstone L (2016) *A Straight Talking Introduction to Psychiatric Diagnosis*. Ross-on-Wye: PCCS Books.

Johnstone L, Boyle M with Cromby J, Dillon J, Harper D, Kinderman P, Longden E, Pilgrim D, Read J (2018). *The Power Threat Meaning Framework: towards the identification of patterns in emotional distress, unusual experiences and troubled or troubling behaviour, as an alternative to functional psychiatric diagnosis*. Leicester: British Psychological Society.

Read J, Bentall RP, Fosse R (2009). Time to abandon the bio-bio-bio model of psychosis: exploring the epigenetic and psychological mechanisms by which adverse life events lead to psychotic symptoms. *Epidemiologia e Psichiatria Sociale 18*: 299–310.

Sanders P (2017). Principled and strategic opposition to the medicalisation of distress and all its apparatus. In: Joseph S (ed). *The Handbook of Person-Centred Therapy and Mental Health: theory, research and practice*. Monmouth: PCCS Books; 2017 (pp11–36).

Stevens E (2019). *The medicalisation of therapy – what we can infer from the language of ScoPEd*. A Client First; 25 June. https://aclientfirst.com/2019/06/25/the-medicalisation-of-therapy-what-can-we-infer-from-the-language-of-scoped/ (accessed 29 June 2019).

Time to Change (2017). *'I was born with OCD and it's part of me.'* [Online.] Time to Change; 28 June. www.time-to-change.org.uk/blog/i-was-born-ocd-and-its-part-me (accessed 29 June 2019).

Wilkinson R, Pickett K (2018). *The Inner Level: how more equal societies reduce stress, restore sanity and improve everyone's well-being*. London: Allen Lane.

Wilkinson R, Pickett K (2010). *The Spirit Level: why greater equality makes societies stronger*. London: Bloomsbury Press.

World Health Organization (2018). *International Classification of Diseases* (11th revision). Geneva: WHO.

Reading and resources

Books

Bentall RP (2009). *Doctoring the Mind: why psychiatric treatments fail.* London: Allen Lane/Penguin.

Breggin PR (1993). *Toxic Psychiatry.* London: Fontana.

Caplan PJ (1995). *They Say You're Crazy: how the world's most powerful psychiatrists decide who's normal.* Reading, MA: Addison Wesley.

Cromby J, Harper D, Reavey P (eds) (2013). *Understanding Mental Health and Distress: beyond abnormal psychology.* Basingstoke: Palgrave Macmillan.

Davies J (2017). *The Sedated Society: the causes and harms of our psychiatric drug epidemic.* Basingstoke: Palgrave Macmillan.

Davies J (2013). *Cracked: why psychiatry is doing more harm than good.* London: Icon Books.

Eaton J, Paterson-Young C (2018). *The Little Orange Book: learning about abuse from the voice of the child.* Staffordshire: VictimFocus.

Fernando S (2002). *Mental Health, Race and Culture* (2nd ed). Basingstoke: Palgrave Macmillan.

Filer N (2019). *The Heartland: finding and losing schizophrenia.* London: Faber & Faber.

Grant A, Biley F, Walker H (2011). *Our Encounters with Madness.* Ross-on-wye: PCCS Books.

Grant A, Haire J, Biley F, Stone B (2017). *Our Encounters with Suicide.* Ross-on-wye: PCCS Books.

Greenberg G (2014). *The Book of Woe: the DSM and the unmaking of psychiatry*. Victoria: Scribe Publications Pty.

Hari J (2018). *Lost Connections: why you're depressed and how to find to hope*. London: Bloomsbury.

Kutchins H (2003). *Making Us Crazy: DSM: the psychiatric bible and the creation of mental disorders*. New York, NY: Free Press.

Healy D (2003). *Let Them Eat Prozac*. Toronto: James Lormier & Co.

Herman JL (2015). *Trauma and Recovery: from domestic abuse to political terror*. New York, NY: Basic Books.

Hunter N (2018). *Trauma and Madness in Mental Health Services*. Basingstoke: Palgrave Macmillan.

Johnstone L (2014). *A Straight Talking Introduction to Psychiatric Diagnosis*. Ross-on-Wye: PCCS Books.

Johnstone L (2000). *Users and Abusers of Psychiatry: a critical look at psychiatric practice* (2nd ed). Hove: Routledge.

Johnstone L, Boyle M, with Cromby J, Dillon J, Harper D, Kinderman P, Longden E, Pilgrim D, Read J (2018). *The Power Threat Meaning Framework: overview*. Leicester: British Psychological Society. This and associated documents are available free from www.bps.org.uk/news-and-policy/introducing-power-threat-meaning-framework

Johnstone L, Dallos R (eds) (2013). *Formulation in Psychology and Psychotherapy: making sense of people's problems* (2nd ed). London: Routledge.

Kinderman P (2019). *A Manifesto for Mental Health: why we need a revolution in mental health care*. Basingstoke: Palgrave Macmillan.

Kinderman P (2014). *A Prescription for Psychiatry*. Basingstoke: Palgrave Macmillan.

Loewenthal D (Ed) (2015). *Critical Psychotherapy, Psychoanalysis and Counselling: implications for practice*. Basingstoke: Palgrave Macmillan.

Lynch T (2014). *Beyond Prozac: healing mental distress*. Ross-on-Wye: PCCS Books.

McFarlane J (2014). *Skydiving for Beginners: a journey of recovery and hope*. Edinburgh: Scottish Independent Advocacy Alliance.

Moncrieff J (2016). *A Straight Talking Introduction to Psychiatric Drugs*. Ross-on-Wye: PCCS Books.

Rapley M, Moncrieff J, Dillon J (eds) (2011). *De-Medicalizing Misery: psychiatry, psychology and the human condition*. Basingstoke: Palgrave Macmillan.

Pilgrim D (2018). *Child Sexual Abuse: moral panic or state of denial?* London: Routledge.

Read J, Dillon J (eds) (2013). *Models of Madness: psychological, social and biological approaches to psychosis* (2nd ed). London: Routledge.

Read J, Sanders P (2010). *A Straight Talking Introduction to the Causes of Mental Health Problems.* Ross-on-Wye: PCCS Books.

Romme M, Escher S, Corstens D, Morris M (2009). *Living with Voices: 50 stories of recovery.* Ross-on-Wye: PCCS Books.

Russo J, Sweeney A (eds) (2016). *Searching for a Rose Garden: challenging psychiatry, fostering mad studies.* Monmouth: PCCS Books.

Sen D (2017). *DSM-69: Dolly Sen's manual of psychiatric disorder.* Newhaven: Eleusinian Press.

Sidley G (2015). *Tales of the Madhouse: an insider critique of psychiatric services.* Ross-on-Wye: PCCS Books.

Van der Kolk B (2014). *The Body Keeps the Score: mind, brain and body in the transformation of trauma.* New York, NY: Viking.

Watters E (2011). *Crazy Like Us: the globalization of the western mind.* London: Constable & Robinson.

Whitaker R (2011). *Anatomy of an Epidemic: magic bullets, psychiatric drugs, and the astonishing rise of mental illness in America.* New York, NY: Crown Publishing Group.

Whitaker R (2010). *Mad in America: bad science, bad medicine, and the enduring mistreatment of the mentally ill.* New York, NY: Basic Books.

Wilkinson R, Pickett K (2018). *The Inner Level: how more equal societies reduce stress, restore sanity and improve everyone's well-being.* London: Penguin.

Useful websites and links

The British Psychological Society, Introducing the Power Threat Meaning Framework – www.bps.org.uk/news-and-policy/introducing-power-threat-meaning-framework

Council for Evidence-Based Psychiatry – www.cepuk.org

A Disorder for Everyone – www.adisorder4everyone.com

A Disorder for Everyone, YouTube channel – www.youtube.com/channel/UCaWG15Tqjo6sZ7obcnKc_Mw

Drop the Disorder Facebook group – www.facebook.com/groups/1182483948461309

Eleanor Longden, *The Voices in My Head*, TED Talk – www.ted.com/talks/eleanor_longden_the_voices_in_my_head

Emerging Proud – www.emergingproud.com

Ending Harm from Psychiatric Diagnosis – www.psychdiagnosis.weebly.com

Gary Sidley's blog – www.talesfromthemadhouse.com

The Icarus Project – www.theicarusproject.net

Inner Compass Initiative – www.theinnercompass.org

Intervoice – The International Hearing Voices Network – www.intervoiceonline.org

Jacqui Dillon website – www.jacquidillon.org

Mad in America – www.madinamerica.com

Mad in the UK – www.madintheuk.com

Paula Joan Caplan website – www.paulajcaplan.net

Philip Hickey website – www.behaviorismandmentalhealth.com

Terry Lynch website – www.doctorterrylynch.com

United for Integrity in Mental Health – www.uimh.org

Contributors

Dr Paula J Caplan
Paula Caplan is a clinical and research psychologist and Associate in the Du Bois Institute of the Hutchins Center for African and African American Research at Harvard University. She has been a Fellow in the Harvard Kennedy School's Women and Public Policy Program. She served for two years on the *DSM-IV* task force before she resigned on moral, ethical, and professional grounds. In addition to her books *They Say You're Crazy: how the world's most powerful psychiatrists decide who's normal* and *Bias in Psychiatric Diagnosis,* she has written a stage play, *CALL ME CRAZY*, which won one of the top prizes in the Arlene and William National Playwriting Contest for Women and had a rave-reviewed Off-Off-Broadway production. She is the author of 10 other books, one of which won three top prizes for non-fiction, and two award-winning documentaries. Paulajcaplan.net and psychdiagnosis.weebly.com

Chris Coombs
Chris Coombs is studying to become a therapist. He is a suicide-attempt survivor who has dealt with depression and anxiety on a personal level for more than a decade. Over that time, he has found those initially helpful labels to be increasingly redundant and has come to focus more on personal identity and meaning. He has recently begun blogging about his experience of internalised able-ism and taboos from within the disability community, at memyselfanddisability.wordpress.com

Dr James Davies
James Davies graduated from the University of Oxford in 2006 with a PhD in social and medical anthropology. He is Reader in Social Anthropology and Mental Health at the University of Roehampton and is also a psychotherapist, having worked with organisations such as Mind and the NHS. He has lectured at universities including Harvard, Yale, Oxford, Oslo, Brown, UCL and Columbia.

He has written articles for the *Times, New Scientist, Guardian* and *Salon*, and has authored and/or edited seven books, including *Cracked: why psychiatry is doing more harm than good* (Icon Books, 2013). He is co-founder of the Council for Evidence-based Psychiatry, which is now secretariat to the All-Party Parliamentary Group for Prescribed Drug Dependence.

Dr Jacqui Dillon

Dr Jacqui Dillon is a writer, activist, international speaker and trainer. She has personal and professional experience, awareness and skills in working with trauma and abuse, dissociation, 'psychosis', hearing voices, healing and recovery. Jacqui has lectured and published worldwide. She is a skilled facilitator in complex learning environments and has a track record of creating and sustaining user-centred initiatives and of affecting change at all levels. Jacqui is also a voice-hearer.

Sally Fox

Sally Fox uses visual arts and the written word to explore and communicate her experience of mental distress and using services. She has performed and exhibited widely, and her work has been published in the *British Journal of Psychiatry* and several poetry anthologies. Her areas of interest include the therapeutic process and relationship, trauma and attachment, art therapy and art journaling, LGBT identities, and the effect of labelling – in particular, 'borderline personality disorder' – around all of which she has devised and facilitated groups and events. She has also contributed to training mental health nurses and other professionals. Sally is passionate about the power of creativity to help us find our authentic voice and use it to influence change. Her books include *Putting Myself in the Frame: drawing hope from art therapy* and (co-authored with Jo McFarlane) *Stigma and Stones: living with a diagnosis of BPD*.

Sue Irwin

Sue Irwin is a keen gardener and linguist, mum to three children, friend and sister. She also sees herself as a survivor of childhood abuse and the UK's mental health system, where she spent 18 years as a service user. Following this, she worked as a paid peer support worker within the NHS, but resigned after 12 months and, shortly after, wrote an article explaining her reasons for leaving. She went on to work in the third sector, facilitating a community volunteer peer support service, and is currently studying for an MSc in social and therapeutic horticulture at Coventry University.

Dr Lucy Johnstone

Dr Lucy Johnstone is a consultant clinical psychologist, author of *Users and Abusers of Psychiatry*, now in its second edition (Routledge, 2000), co-editor of *Formulation in Psychology and Psychotherapy: making sense of people's problems*, also in its second edition (Routledge, 2013), and author of *A Straight-*

Talking Introduction to Psychiatric Diagnosis (PCCS Books, 2014), along with a number of other chapters and articles taking a critical perspective on mental health theory and practice. She is the former programme director of the Bristol Clinical Psychology Doctorate and was the lead author of the Division of Clinical Psychology's *Good Practice Guidelines on the Use of Psychological Formulation* (2011). She has worked in adult mental health settings for many years, most recently in a service in South Wales. She was lead author, with Professor Mary Boyle, of the Power Threat Meaning Framework, a project funded by the Division of Clinical Psychology to outline a conceptual alternative to psychiatric diagnosis, which was published in January 2018. Lucy is an experienced conference speaker and lecturer, and currently works as an independent trainer. Her particular interest and expertise are in the use of psychological formulation, in both its individual and team versions, and in promoting trauma-informed practice.

Professor Peter Kinderman
Peter Kinderman is Professor of Clinical Psychology at the University of Liverpool and former President of the British Psychological Society. Peter's focus is on transformational change in how we understand 'mental health', and therefore on the reform of mental health services. His research interests are in psychological processes underpinning wellbeing and mental health. He has published widely on the role of psychological factors as mediators between biological, social and circumstantial factors in mental health and wellbeing, and has received significant research grant funding – most recently from the Economic and Social Research Council (ESRC), to lead a three-year evidence synthesis programme for the What Works Centre for Wellbeing, exploring the effectiveness of policies aimed at improving community wellbeing, and from the National Institute for Health Research to investigate the effectiveness of human rights training in dementia care. His most recent book, *A Manifesto for Mental Health* (Palgrave Macmillan, 2019), presents his vision for the future of mental health services. You can follow him on Twitter @peterkinderman

Guilaine Kinouani
Guilaine Kinouani is a feminist, equality consultant, therapist and award-nominated writer. Her analyses are rooted in her social location as a Black French woman, a migrant and a (proud) child of the Banlieue, with solid roots in Africa. She is currently completing her doctorate in clinical psychology. You can read some of her writing at www.racereflections.co.uk

Dr Terry Lynch
Terry Lynch is a medical doctor, psychotherapist, mental health educator and mental health author. Mental health has been his special interest for the past 30 years. Having worked as a GP for 10 years, by the late 1990s he had lost faith in the medical approach to mental health. He retrained as a psychotherapist

and has been providing a recovery-oriented mental health service in Ireland for the past 20 years. Most people who consult him have already been given a psychiatric diagnosis. Terry's priorities include a) the dismantling of the fundamentally flawed medical (mis)understanding of mental health, and b) the widespread adoption of a far more accurate understanding that is trauma-informed, recovery-oriented and contains effective and accessible pathways towards healing and recovery. Terry Lynch has been appointed to several Irish national mental health groups, including the Expert Group on Mental Health Policy (2003–06), which formulated *A Vision for Change,* Ireland's official mental health policy document. Terry is also a founder member of United for Integrity in Mental Health (UIMH). www.doctorterrylynch.com

Dr Lorenza Magliano

Lorenza Magliano is Associate Professor of Psychiatry at the Department of Psychology of the Campania University 'Luigi Vanvitelli', Caserta (Italy). Her main research fields cover burden, coping strategies and social networks in mental health and physical disorders; stigma against people with 'psychosis' and other mental health problems; educational interventions to reduce prejudices about people with 'psychosis' among future health professionals, and development and implementation of psychosocial interventions for people experiencing severe emotional distress and their families in routine settings. She is co-author of about 80 scientific papers in peer-reviewed journals, and of the Italian handbook on psychiatric rehabilitation, *Valutazione delle Abilità e Definizione degli Obiettivi (VADO)* (*Skills Assessment and Definition of Goals*) (Edizione Erickson, 1998). She is also among the contributors to the books *Experiencing Psychosis* (Routledge, 2012), and *Models of Madness: psychological, social and biological approaches to psychosis* (2nd edition; Routledge, 2013). She is a member of the editorial board of the journal *Psychosis* and of the scientific board of the Italian Society of Psychiatric Epidemiology.

Professor John Read

John Read is Professor of Clinical Psychology at the University of East London. John worked for nearly 20 years as a clinical psychologist and manager of mental health services in the UK and the US, before joining the University of Auckland, New Zealand, in 1994, where he worked until 2013. He has published more than 130 papers in research journals, primarily on the relationship between adverse life events (eg. child abuse/neglect, poverty etc) and 'psychosis'. He also researches the negative effects of bio-genetic causal explanations on prejudice, the opinions and experiences of recipients of antipsychotic and antidepressant medication, and the role of the pharmaceutical industry in mental health research and practice. John is on the Executive Committee of the International Society for Psychological and Social Approaches to Psychosis (www.isps.org) and is the editor of the ISPS's scientific journal, *Psychosis*.

Pete Sanders

Pete Sanders spent over 35 years practising as a counsellor, educator and clinical supervisor when he was the course leader on three BACP-recognised courses and was centrally involved in establishing and running the BACP Trainer Accreditation Scheme. He founded PCCS Books with Maggie, his wife, in 1993 and has written, co-written and edited numerous books, chapters and papers on many aspects of counselling, psychotherapy and mental health. He has given keynote addresses at several UK and European conferences and continues to have active interests in developing person-centred theory, the politics of counselling and psychotherapy and the de-medicalisation of distress. He is a pre-therapy/contact work trainer, patron of the Soteria Network UK and trustee of Open Door Counselling, Birmingham. He is trying to retire.

Dolly Sen

Dolly Sen is a writer, film-maker, mental health consultant and trainer, with lived experience of 'psychosis', 'mood disorder' and 'PTSD'. Her training and public speaking has taken her to the World Health Organization in Geneva, Oxford University, the Barbican, Mayor of London, University of Westminster, Guy's Hospital, the Probation Service and more than 100 charity, corporate and statutory organisations. She has written more than 10 books and contributed chapters to more than 20 others, and she has made more than 30 media appearances on TV, radio, internet and in print. Her other mental health work involves consultancy, keynote speaking, coaching, research, group facilitation, campaigning, social media and creative work.

Clare Shaw

Described by the Arvon Foundation as 'one of the country's most dynamic young poets', Clare Shaw has three collections published with Bloodaxe – *Straight Ahead* (2006), which attracted a Forward Prize Highly Commended for Best Single Poem; *Head On* (2012), which the *Times Literary Supplement* called 'fierce… memorable and visceral', and *Flood* (2018). Clare was born in Burnley in 1972, and her poetry finds its roots in place and an uncompromising voice. Her poetry often addresses political and personal conflict and it is fuelled by a strong conviction in the transformative and redemptive power of language. Clare is an Associate Fellow with the Royal Literary Fund, and a regular tutor with the Poetry School, the Wordsworth Trust, the National Writer's Centre of Wales and the Arvon Foundation. She is also a mental health trainer, activist and author. Recent publications include *Otis Doesn't Scratch: talking to young children about self-injury* (PCCS Books, 2015) and (as co-editor) *Our Encounters with Self-Harm* (PCCS Books, 2013).

Dr Gary Sidley

Gary worked in NHS mental health services for 33 years in a variety of nursing, psychological and managerial roles. In the 1980s he was employed as a psychiatric nurse at a large asylum in Manchester. He began his clinical psychology training in 1987 and subsequently worked as a clinical psychologist in community mental health services, inpatient units and GP practices, as well as a professional lead and a member of an NHS trust's senior management team. Gary opted for early retirement in 2013 and currently is a freelance writer and trainer with an interest in promoting alternatives to biomedical psychiatry as ways of responding to human suffering. He writes on a range of topics, including alternatives to biological psychiatry (his book, *Tales from the Madhouse: an insider critique of psychiatric services*, was published by PCCS Books in 2015); general-interest articles, and humour. Gary is also a moderator of the Drop the Disorder! Facebook group.

Jenny Taper

Jenny Taper is a counsellor, supervisor and tutor with more than 10 years' experience of working with young people, adults, couples, families and groups. She has worked in schools, family centres, employment support services and private practice. The majority of clients she has worked with have experienced trauma and abuse, and many have also been given a psychiatric diagnosis. As a tutor, she ensured that her students understood the difficulties of working within the current system, where, in many settings, services are only accessible to those in receipt of a diagnosis, alongside teaching them to challenge the prevailing narrative of 'disorder'. Following a relocation to Cornwall, she is now working as a therapist for an occupational health company.

Dr Akima Thomas OBE

Akima Thomas is a feminist activist and comes from a background in nursing and social work. She is founder and Clinical Director of Women and Girls Network, a holistic therapeutic service working with women and girls surviving gendered violence. Akima has pioneered working from a trauma-informed approach and has developed a strengths-based, non-pathologising clinical model, the Holistic Empowerment Recovery model (HER), which integrates healing of mind, body and spirit. More recently, Akima has researched women's healing journeys, chronicling their strategies of resistance, rebellion and resilience to ensure survival.

Lisa Thompson

Lisa Thompson is Chief Executive of the Rape and Sexual Violence Project (RSVP), having worked for them since 1999. RSVP is Birmingham and Solihull's rape crisis charity, national award winners, and in 2018 celebrated its 40th year. RSVP provides children and adults of all genders with hope and confidence after sexual trauma. Lisa qualified as a social worker at Birmingham University in 1992 and has lived in the city ever since. She has 27 years' experience of supporting survivors of sexual violence and abuse. Lisa's grandmother, Gina, survived rape as a teenager and didn't tell anyone for the best part of 70 years. Her grandmother is the reason that Lisa is so passionate about her work.

Robyn Timoclea

Robyn Timoclea is a survivor researcher and anti-'personality disorder' activist with a specialist interest in emancipatory and feminist approaches to distress. She is a member of the anti-'personality disorder' activist group PDintheBin, and has previously facilitated sexual violence and complex needs groups in prisons. Her current research explores the extent to which experiences of traumatised women in forensic services are pathologised. In addition, Robyn has had her own lived experience of surviving sexual violence and a 'personality disorder' diagnosis.

Jamie-Lee Tipping

Jamie-Lee Tipping is currently working as a therapist for an occupational health company. He previously worked for three years as the course leader on a counselling degree at a nationally recognised university. He is a qualified integrative counsellor who has practised for eight years. Jamie-Lee's background is working as a clinical lead in the welfare sector, where he established a successful national counselling service that offers one-to-one and group support for job seekers experiencing emotional distress. His educational background includes various counselling specialisms, including working with couples and supervision. He also has a private practice in Birmingham.

Professor Emmy van Deurzen

Emmy van Deurzen is a philosopher and counselling psychologist, has been an existential psychotherapist for 45 years, and has founded and directed a number of training organisations. She is the Principal of the New School of Psychotherapy and Counselling at the Existential Academy in London, and a visiting professor with Middlesex University. Among her 17 books are *Existential Psychotherapy and Counselling in Practice*, now in its third edition (Sage, 2012), *Psychotherapy and the Quest for Happiness* (Sage, 2009) and *Everyday Mysteries* (2nd edition) (Routledge, 2010). Her second edition of *Paradox and Passion in Psychotherapy* was published by Wiley in 2015.

Jo Watson

Jo Watson (@dropthedisorder) is a psychotherapist and activist with a history in the UK Rape Crisis movement of the 1990s. She has worked therapeutically for the last 24 years with people who have been victims of sexual abuse/violence and has campaigned on women's survivor issues for the past three decades. Jo actively challenges the biomedical model of 'mental health', arguing that emotional distress and suffering are primarily a result of what people have experienced, which all too often arises within social injustices that need to be named. Jo is the organiser, with Dr Lucy Johnstone, of the 'A Disorder For Everyone!' one-day events (www.adisorder4everyone.com) (AD4E). AD4E platforms a growing team of allies, both professionals and survivors, from around the UK and beyond.

It is currently in its third year of touring the UK, challenging the 'diagnosis and disorder' approach. Jo started the Facebook group 'Drop the Disorder!' in 2016 to offer a space for people to discuss related issues and (as of June 2019) it has more than 8,500 members worldwide (https://bit.ly/2vUV2dL). She is part of the Mad in the UK team (www.madintheuk.com) and a founder member of United for Integrity in Mental Health (UIMH).

Becky Willetts

Becky qualified as a social worker in 2009, after completing an initial degree in psychology and drama, then went on to take the post-qualifying award in social work in 2014. Becky has worked in the voluntary sector for most of her career and almost exclusively since qualifying as a social worker. The majority of her experience includes assessment and therapeutic social work. Becky has created and delivered training across a number of areas, to many different audiences, including professionals, foster carers and colleagues. Outside of work, Becky is a keen knitter and cup-of-tea enthusiast.

Name index

Subject index